To Gently Leave This Life
The Right To Die

ELAINE FEUER

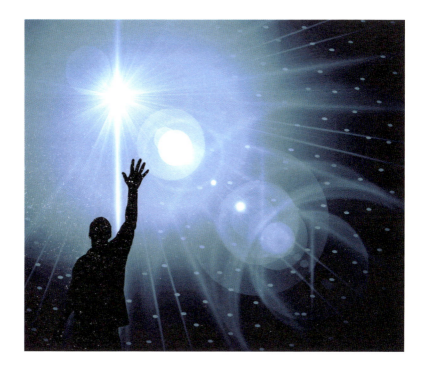

For life and death are one, even as the river and the sea are one...

Kahlil Gibran

Watching a peaceful death of a human being reminds us of a falling star; one of a million lights in a vast sky that flares up for a brief moment only to disappear into the endless night forever.

Elisabeth Kübler-Ross

What Book Reviewers Are Saying!

To Gently Leave This Life is an excellent handbook for those who are living through the struggle now, and those new to the fight who are just realizing what could be in store for them when there is no way out of a prolonged, agonizing death. Elaine Feuer has succeeded in compiling the progress of the Right-To-Die movement in her carefully researched, helpfully illustrated, easily read short volume. This overview explains, especially to the naïve reader, what the human tragedies were that precipitated changes in the law toward further control by patients to control their own deaths. She presents the safeguards and the modest use of these laws to reduce suffering at the end of life and the arguments against these changes. Feuer has worked assiduously to make her information as accurate as possible, to demonstrate the importance of people being able to have more say about when and how the end will come.

Faye Girsh, President
World Federation of Right to Die Societies

An excellent way to help spread the word about the Right-To-Die movement. Another good way is to join the Final Exit Network and get involved. The few of us that feel strongly about having a free choice in determining how much suffering we are willing to tolerate, should be writing letters to the media and doing everything we can to fight the religious right who wish to impose their beliefs on us.

Ken Leonard – *Final Exit Network*

To Gently Leave This Life is an excellent representation of a huge crisis, leaving me with an understanding and urgency to take action, or to somehow make end-of-life decisions more visible to humanity. A very powerful and moving book. At times I had tears and could feel the pain and the plea for compassion from these people, who are either terminally ill or suffering from an incurable disease. All of these voices not heard from, but crying in anguish all the same. Elaine Feuer thoroughly covers the facts and situations of real people, expressed objectively yet profoundly, with information anyone can relate to and understand. It is time to help humanity with this heartfelt book, which needs to be brought into the light and to readers all over the world.

Erna Grinjesch – ***EG's Reality Press***, **NYC**

To Gently Leave This Life is a real eye-opener, as it paves the way for choice and dignity at the end of life. The reader cannot help but ask, "What if it were me?" And if you were diagnosed with ALS, like Sue Rodriguez and Gloria Taylor, and forced to endure a disease that is absolutely terrifying, would you really want to live to the last agonizing minute? Gloria Taylor testified, "I fear that I will eventually suffocate and die struggling for air like a fish out of water." As the assisted death debate expands and intensifies across the globe, I highly recommend ***To Gently Leave This Life*** as a well-researched, timely, and prescient book.

Nora Begley – ***The Southfield Gazette***

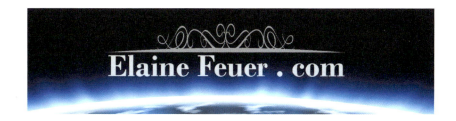

About The Author

Elaine Feuer began contemplating end-of-life issues after witnessing her mother's slow and painful death from cancer. ***To Gently Leave This Life*** is the perfect reference book for the grassroots activist, legislator, and for people who are dealing with their own or a loved one's terminal illness. It is Elaine's aspiration that medical aid in dying will be approved throughout the U.S., Canada, and in other countries. Whenever possible, people deserve the right to have a "gentle and happy" death.

Elaine wrote the critically acclaimed expose, ***Innocent Casualties: The FDA's War Against Humanity***, which is available with 2012 Updates at *http://www.elainefeuer.com*.

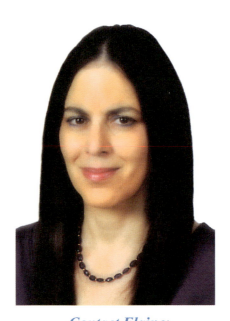

Contact Elaine:

elaine@elainefeuer.com

Author's Note & Copyright

To Gently Leave This Life is a critical review of end-of-life options. It makes no recommendations about medical care. People reading this book must take full responsibility for their own health care. Accordingly, the author and publisher disclaim responsibility for decisions based on information contained herein.

ISBN # 978-0-9889691-6-2

Printed in the United States of America

Designed by Kelly Christen

First Printing

To order additional books, or to contact the author,

go to http://www.elainefeuer.com

elaine@elainefeuer.com

DEDICATION

To all of the extraordinary people who have fought for the right to gently leave this life, in the most difficult of times, during their own or a loved one's illness.

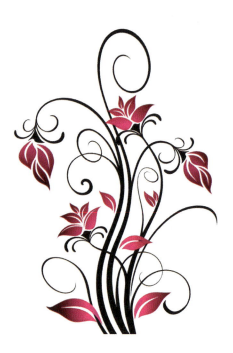

ACKNOWLEDGEMENTS

My appreciation and thanks to Allan Feuer, Sharon Fox, and Anna Grinjesch, for their love, support, and encouragement throughout the duration of this project. Rob Katzman and Larry Kaplan offered their assistance the instant I needed it. I am indebted to Sean Crowley, for making corrections in the manuscript. A big "thank you" to my friends in Vancouver – Dr. Doug Kuramoto, Robin, Bonnie and Rand Blanchette, AKA Randini Martini – for his boundless gifts of love, consolation, and abiding humor. I especially want to thank Hazel and Irwin Hundert – my parents' best friends – for their love and support during my mother's illness and death.

Elaine Feuer
March 2014

Table of Contents

Introduction

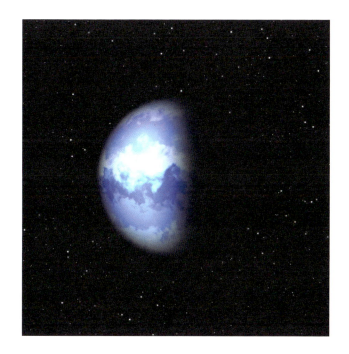

His pain was too great. He begged me for the simple mercy of death. And I could do nothing else but help him leave a world that had become a sleepless, tortured nightmare to him.

Robert D. Andrews

The concept of a "good death" has been debated since the beginning of civilization. In the 21st century, longer lifespans and advances in medicine have resulted in new legislation regarding an individual's "right to die." The option to end one's own life, when pain becomes intolerable or the quality of life is nonexistent, is an issue at the forefront of modern society. Who among us would trade places with a patient, dependent on machines and other people, for every aspect of their life? Who among us wouldn't choose medical aid in dying, if that option were available?

During the last two decades, the states of Oregon, Washington, and Montana have passed Death With Dignity laws, and in the Netherlands, Belgium, and Luxembourg, voluntary euthanasia laws were approved.* However, in 2012, two court cases examining physician aid in dying could lead to new international precedents: Gloria Taylor, who suffered from Lou Gehrig's disease, became the first person in Canada to be granted the "right to die" via a "personal exemption" by British Columbia's Supreme Court; in Britain, Tony Nicklinson, who suffered from "locked-in syndrome" and could only communicate by blinking, died from pneumonia after refusing food and fluids subsequent to a High Court decision that refused to grant him assisted death.

In this age of medical technology, of machines sustaining lives irrespective of quality of life and dignity, we often discount the concept of a "good death." Allowing terminally ill people to pass on quickly and peacefully does not encroach on the civil liberties of others. Aid in dying legislation allows patients to operate within the medical system and ease their anxiety, while giving friends and family peace of mind. Assessing the quality of life, and allowing patients who suffer from debilitating pain and dependence on others to gently leave this life, gives people a dignified alternative.

In a democratic society, the right to choose, the option of free will, is tantamount for survival. In the United States, we value our freedom above all else. We value the right to self-determination and opposing viewpoints. We value life, and we are all mortal.

****

*On May 20th, 2013, Vermont's state legislature voted for aid in dying, and Governor Peter Shumlin signed the bill into law, making Vermont the fourth state to have Death With Dignity laws. In January 2014, a district court in New Mexico authorized doctors to provide lethal prescriptions, declaring it a constitutional right for "a competent, terminally ill patient to choose aid in dying."

Prologue

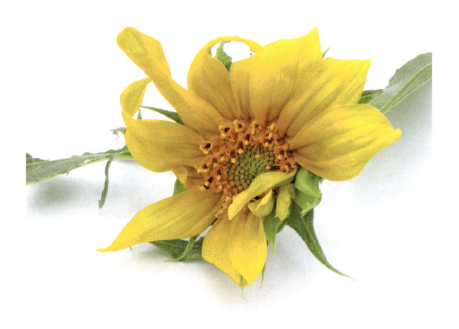

To live in the hearts we leave behind is not to die.

Thomas Campbell

I walked into her hospital room on a sunny Saturday morning, as nurses treated an inflamed bedsore and she grimaced in pain. One of the nurses saw the look on my face and explained that the medication in her IV did not assuage the sting of an open wound. My mother, so thin that her eyes appeared to be bulging, looked up and never took her eyes off of me.

A few minutes later, she leaned forward as I attempted to give her some water from a small paper cup. The water had barely touched her lips when she began to choke, and that same nurse told me that she didn't need fluids since her body was starting to shut down. My mother was too weak to speak – her voice had barely been audible for weeks – but she had moved her head forward, indicating that she wanted the water. So I picked up a small stick with a tiny sponge on one end, dipped the sponge in water, and gently inserted it into her mouth. I pulled up a chair next to her bed, took her hand in mine, and she never took her eyes off of me, and barely, if ever, blinked.

A few hours later, I stepped outside of her room to talk to one of the nurses, who told me that the medical staff thought she had a few more days to live, and asked if I wanted the staff to arrange a hospice vigil. I declined the offer since my mother was a private person and did not want strangers sitting in her room, watching her die. It had been a year since she was told that her breast cancer from five years earlier had returned and metastasized to her left lung and left heart lining, and that this time, the cancer was irreversible. She had told her beloved naturopath, Dr. Doug – who had saved her life in 2002 – that what she feared the most was losing her dignity, and that she "wasn't going to sit around, waiting to die." Doug looked at her without saying anything for such a long time that she finally asked him what he was thinking about and he told her, "I was just thinking how much I love you."

She had been expected to live for only a few months, but I was not surprised that she hung on for another year. A hospital procedure - draining the fluid in her left lung and connecting her left lung lining to her left rib, to stop the build-up of fluid - was very hard on her, but the procedure prolonged her life. Just when it seemed, on many of those endless days when she could barely get out of bed, that the end might be near, she would rally, waking up the next morning and acting as if she were perfectly healthy.

She was such a Spartan, insisting on doing almost everything herself, even when it was painful and hard to do, because she needed to accomplish things, whether it was washing the dishes or walking in pain to the car, instead of letting me drive to the back door of the apartment building to pick her up. She would never acknowledge that she was in pain, and the nurses who came to the apartment, as well as her doctors, didn't realize how much pain she was in because they would see her sitting in a chair, wearing a lovely peach sweater and pearl earrings – but that's what she was like her entire life. The last thing she wanted was for anyone to feel sorry for her, and that was very hard for me, knowing that she was in worse shape than she disclosed. Her doctors and nurses tried to ask her what her pain level was, from 0 – no pain, to 10 – extreme pain – but they finally gave up asking that question because she would never answer it with specificity – she always said that she was fine.

On that last weekend at home, she had to lean against the wall in order to not fall; she became delirious and stopped making sense; and she forgot to turn off a burner on the gas stove. Monday morning, her doctor sent an ambulance to the apartment, and when she woke up after that first night in the hospital, and was frightened because she didn't know where she was, I decided to stay with her in her hospital room for the rest of the week. During that last year of her life, when cancer indiscriminately ravaged her physical, mental, and emotional wellbeing, she only felt safe when she was with me.

It was those last seven weeks in the hospital that were the most difficult and heartbreaking, watching her suffer, watching as her face and body became emaciated, pretending that I understood what she was saying when I did not. Her foremost concern had been to preserve her dignity, yet it was taken away from her, hour-by-hour, day-by-day.

On that final Saturday evening, snow sparkled through the window and a crackling fire bellowed on the TV screen, giving the illusion of a fireplace in her room. A beautiful warm auburn comforter covered her thin body. I sat in the chair next to her bed, held her hand, and said, "Mom, you can release yourself from this torture." And she blinked twice, which meant, "yes." As we sat in silence, looking at each other, minutes turned into hours. By 5am Sunday morning, her eyes closed for the last time, and her doctor told me that she had passed on. I sat with her for three more hours, sensing that her soul was still in the room with me, comforted that she was still in the room with me. The nurse who had told me the night before that she thought my mother had a few more days to live, rushed over to me to say how relieved she was that I had stayed all night at the hospital, and I wondered if that nurse realized how extraordinary she was, caring so much. Finally, at 8am, I called a few family members and friends, gathered her belongings, and left the hospital for the last time.

Would she have wanted a way out, earlier than those seven weeks in the hospital? A few days before she died, her voice suddenly became audible again and she kept demanding, over and over, "I want to go home! I want to go home! I want to go home!" until she exhausted herself and could do nothing on her own, ever again. I am certain that, given the choice, she would have asked for doctor-assisted help, to go peacefully into the night, rather than spend seven excruciating weeks in the hospital.

What she had wanted more than anything, what worried her the most, was maintaining her dignity. She had signed a DNR requesting "Do Not Resuscitate" but that alone, did not free her from pain or ensure her dignity. I didn't think it was asking too much for her to pass on in her own bed, in her own home. It wasn't asking too much to end the suffering she was forced to endure in the hospital. All she wanted was her dignity, and that wasn't asking for too much.

CHAPTER ONE

Euthanasia: Early Definitions

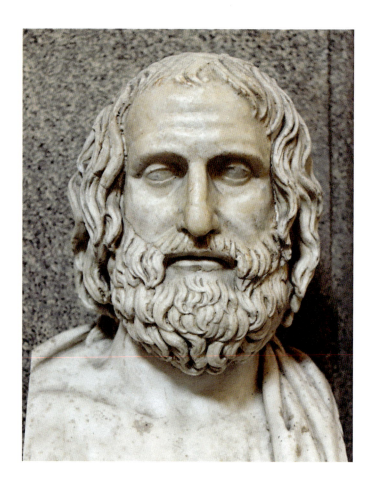

No one can confidently say that he will still be living tomorrow.

Euripides

A Good Death:

Voluntary euthanasia or physician-assisted death comes from the Greek words "eu" and "thanatos" and means "a good death" or "a gentle and easy death" – the intentional ending of a life when the patient is suffering from a terminal illness or an incurable disease.

Early Definition of Euthanasia:

The word "euthanasia" comes from a historian's description of Roman Emperor Augustus's death (19 August AD 14), one month before his 76th birthday: He "died quickly and without suffering in the arms of his wife, Livia, experiencing the 'euthanasia' he had wished for."

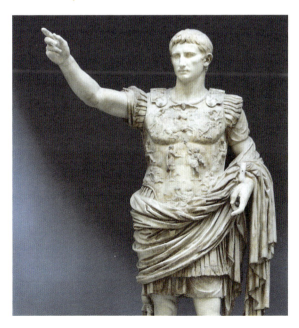

Roman Emperor Augustus

Euthanasia in a Medical Context:

In the 17th Century, the English philosopher, Francis Bacon, defined euthanasia in a medical context, as a "physician's responsibility to alleviate the physical sufferings of the body" for an easy, painless, and happy death."

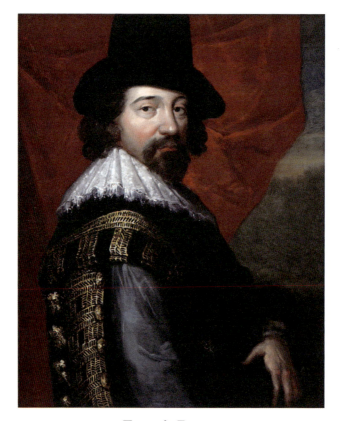

Francis Bacon

In modern society, euthanasia refers to a painless death, such as a lethal injection, for people who are suffering from a terminal or incurable disease.

Intent:

The intent of euthanasia is to alleviate intolerable suffering by providing a merciful death.

Four Types of Euthanasia:

1) **Active or Voluntary Euthanasia** occurs when a patient asks for a lethal injection.
2) **Non-Voluntary Euthanasia** occurs when the consent of the patient is unattainable, such as when a patient is in a coma.
3) **Involuntary Euthanasia** occurs when a patient is removed from medical support against their will.
4) **Passive Euthanasia** occurs when a treatment to prolong life is withheld, such as antibiotics for a terminally ill patient with pneumonia.

Euthanasia Arguments, Pro and Con:

In the 21st Century, euthanasia advocates contend that:

1) People have a right to self-determination and a right to choose their own fate;
2) Helping a person to die is preferable to insisting that they continue to suffer;
3) The distinction between passive and active euthanasia is not necessarily important;
4) Euthanasia does not have negative consequences.

In the 21st Century, euthanasia opponents contend that:

1) Deaths are not necessarily painful;
2) Treatments do not have to be "active" – such as giving terminally ill patients antibiotics for pneumonia. Instead of the antibiotics, the patient is given adequate pain medication to die peacefully. For this reason, pneumonia is often referred to as "the old person's friend";
3) The distinction between active and passive euthanasia is important;
4) Legalizing euthanasia is a "slippery slope" with adverse consequences.

CHAPTER TWO

History Of Euthanasia

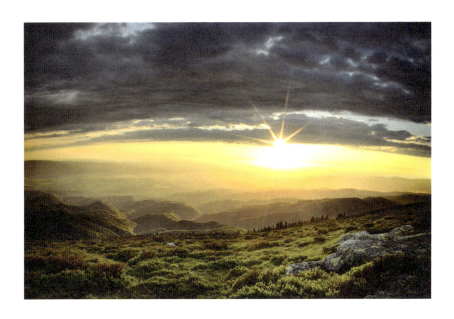

The ancients stressed the voluntary nature of dying, provided that it was done for the right reasons... to end the suffering of a terminal illness.

Michael Manning, M.D.

Ancient Greece and Rome

5th Century B.C. - 1st Century B.C.:

Euthanasia was an approved practice in Ancient Greece and Rome. Socrates, Plato, Roman essayist Marcus Annaeus Seneca, as well as other notables, sanctioned the use of Hemlock, to hasten a person's death. Although the Hippocratic Oath prohibited doctors from giving "a deadly drug to anybody, not even if asked for," most Greek and Roman physicians did not comply with the oath.

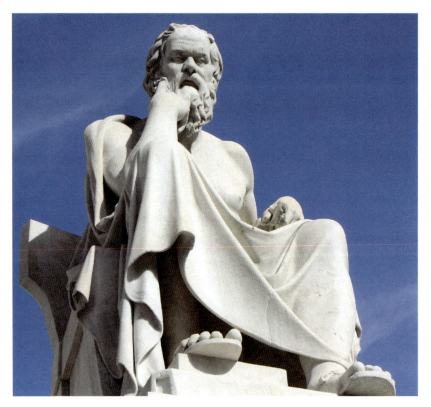

Socrates

The Age of Faith

1st Century A.D. - Late Middle Ages:

Judeo-Christian philosophy was in direct opposition to euthanasia. St. Thomas Aquinas argued that assisted death conflicted with man's survival instincts. Islam teachings also impart that God is the Creator and that only God may take life away.

17th Century:

Common law tradition prohibited suicide and assisted death in the American Colonies.

The Age of Enlightenment

Renaissance and Reformation in the 17th - 18th Century:

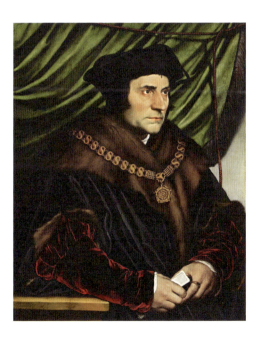

Thomas More

Writers challenged the authority of the church and supported euthanasia, denoting Thomas More's *Utopia* (1516), which envisioned a civilization that expedited the passing for those experiencing a slow and torturous death.

18th Century - American Evangelical Christians:

Euthanasia was condemned in the earliest days of the 13 Colonies.

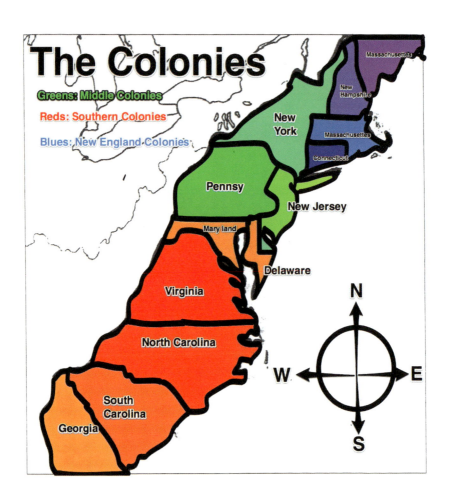

1828 - First American Statute to Outlaw Assisted Death in New York:

A New York commission drafted a criminal code that prohibited assisted death, and many of the new States and Territories followed New York's example.

1870s - Morphine Used for Euthanasia:

Samuel Williams advocated widespread use of analgesics for euthanasia, and the issue was examined in thought-provoking articles in medical and scientific journals.

1894 - Euthanasia and Terminal Illnesses:

Robert Ingersoll, known as *The Great Agnostic*, argued that people suffering from a terminal illness, such as cancer, had the right to legalized euthanasia.

Early 20th Century - U.S. Hospital System:

The first phase of a nation-wide hospital system coincided with the emergence of the euthanasia debate in the early 20th Century.

1906 - Euthanasia Bill Defeated in Ohio:

Henry Hunt attempted to have euthanasia legalized in Ohio. His bill supported people in agonizing pain and/or with a terminal illness.

1930s - Support For Euthanasia Increases During Great Depression:

Forty-five percent of Americans supported the mercy killing of infants born physically or mentally handicapped, with no possible cure.

1935 - National Society for the Legalization of Euthanasia (VELS) in England:

C.K. Millard, a public health physician, founded the VELS.

1938 - National Society for the Legalization of Euthanasia (NSLE) in U.S.:

Charles Francis Potter founded the NSLE - later renamed the Euthanasia Society of America - ESA. Members of the ESA supported physician-assisted death for people with incurable diseases. Its trustees included Dr. Clarence Cook, with the American Society for the Control of Cancer and the American Birth Control League, and Secretary Leon Fradley Whitney, with the American Eugenics Society.

1940s - Nazi Use of "Involuntary Euthanasia" or Mass Murder, Changes American Perceptions of Euthanasia:

In the late 1930s and early 1940s, it appeared as if euthanasia would soon be legal in the U.S. However, Americans opposed to euthanasia compared the Nazi atrocities against its own citizens to pro-euthanasia advocates in the U.S.

The Nazi "euthanasia campaign" was a euphemism for mass murder: The agenda was genocide, for those with disabilities, dissenting political, or dissenting religious beliefs. More than 70,000 German citizens were killed in gas vans and "killing centers."

The foundation of "Nazi euthanasia" pre-dated Hitler and the Third Reich, and was connected to eugenics – selective breeding – and to social Darwinism – "survival of the fittest." Nazi euthanasia was based on *The Right to Death*, published in 1895. Its author, Adolf Jost, maintained that the state – the "social organism" – controls the individual, thereby giving the state the right to control or euthanize the death of the individual. The state must kill in order to keep the "social organism" healthy, and the individual's rights regarding death are dependent on the individual's fitness for life.

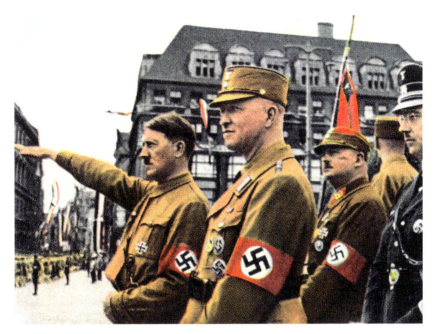

Adolf Hitler and the Third Reich

1946 - Committee of 1776 Physicians for Legalizing Voluntary Euthanasia Founded in New York.

1965 - Donald McKinney, President of Euthanasia Society of America (ESA):

Donald McKinney transformed the euthanasia movement by making a distinction between active and passive euthanasia. He became a forerunner in the euthanasia debate and led a sizable group of people who opposed active euthanasia.

1967 - Living Will:

Attorney Luis Kutner wrote the first living will. His arguments were published in the *Indiana Law Journal*.

1974 - Society for the "Right to Die" Founded:

The Society for the "Right to Die" [formerly the Euthanasia Society of America] was founded. It supported the legalization of active euthanasia, and campaigned for it via the political process.

1974 - First U.S. Hospice:

The first American hospice opened in New Haven, Connecticut.

1976 - Karen Quinlan Legal Case:

On Mar. 31, 1976, the Supreme Court ruled that a respirator could be removed from coma patients.

(See Chapter Six - Karen Quinlan: The Right To Die)

1980 - World Federation of "Right to Die" Societies Founded:

In 1980, the World Federation of "Right to Die" Societies was created, and its membership included organizations from several countries.

1980 - Hemlock Society:

Derek Humphry, one of the innovators in the American euthanasia movement, started the Hemlock Society, a grassroots euthanasia organization in Los Angeles that supported active euthanasia – physician-assisted death.

1988 - Journal of the American Medical Association (JAMA) Publishes Article By Hospital Worker Who Euthanized a Patient:

In 1988, *JAMA* published an anonymous article describing how a doctor in residence injected a patient – who was suffering from ovarian cancer – with an overdose of morphine, to put the patient out of pain. "It's Over Debbie" caused the expected controversy and helped to ignite the debate about physician-assisted death.

1990s - Public Opinion Surveys: More Than 50 Percent of Americans Support Medical Aid In Dying:

By the 1990s, public interest in the "right to die" movement increased. Public opinion surveys demonstrated that more than 50 percent of Americans supported physician-assisted death. Membership of the Hemlock Society increased to 50,000, and the rise of public interest increased voluntary euthanasia activity in the courts, in professional medical journals, and in institutions.

1994 - Oregon "Death With Dignity Act" Approved:

For the first time in U.S. history, medical aid in dying became legal in an American state via the legislative process.

(See Chapter 11 - Oregon, Washington, Montana: Death With Dignity Laws)

1997 - U.S. Supreme Court Rules "Right to Die" is Unconstitutional:

The Supreme Court ruled in *Glucksberg v. Washington* and *Vacco v. Quill*, that the "right to die" is unconstitutional.

1997 - Oregon Votes to Keep "Death With Dignity Act":

(See Chapter 11 - Oregon, Washington, Montana: Death With Dignity Laws)

1998 - Dr. Jack Kevorkian Performs Voluntary Euthanasia on National Television and is Convicted of Murder in 1999:

(See Chapter 9 - Dr. Jack Kevorkian: Hero or Criminal?)

2001 - Netherlands Legalizes Voluntary Euthanasia:

(See Chapter 12 - Netherlands, Belgium, Luxembourg: Voluntary Euthanasia Laws)

2002 - Belgium Legalizes Voluntary Euthanasia:

(See Chapter 12 - Netherlands, Belgium, Luxembourg: Voluntary Euthanasia Laws)

2003 - Bush Administration Challenges Oregon's "Death with Dignity" Legislation:

U.S. Attorney-General John Ashcroft asked the 9th Circuit Court of Appeals to reverse the findings of a lower court that legalized the Oregon "Death With Dignity Act" of 1994, claiming that it infringed on federal powers.

(See Chapter 11 - Oregon, Washington, Montana: Death With Dignity Laws)

2005 - Compassion and Choices: "Compassion in Dying" and "End-of-Life Choices" unite, becoming the largest organization in the U.S. that advocates for patients' rights at the end of life.

2005 - Terri Schiavo's Feeding Tube Removed:

(See Chapter 7 - Terri Schiavo: Vegetative State)

2006 - U.S. Supreme Court Upholds Oregon's "Death With Dignity Act":

In a 6-3 decision, the Supreme Court stated that the federal Attorney General did not have the right to challenge Oregon's "Death with Dignity Act." *Gonzales v. Oregon*, Jan. 17, 2006.

(See Chapter 11 - Oregon, Washington, Montana: Death With Dignity Laws)

2008 - Luxembourg Legalizes Voluntary Euthanasia:

(See Chapter 12 - Netherlands, Belgium, Luxembourg: Voluntary Euthanasia Laws)

2009 - State of Washington Legalizes Death With Dignity Act:

(See Chapter 11 - Oregon, Washington, Montana: Death With Dignity Laws)

2009 - State of Montana Legalizes Aid in Dying:

(See Chapter 11 - Oregon, Washington, Montana: Death With Dignity Laws)

2012 - Massachusetts "Death with Dignity" Ballot Measure Defeated.

2013 – Vermont's State Legislature Passes Aid In Dying Bill, Making Vermont the Fourth State to have Death With Dignity Laws.

2014 – New Mexico Authorizes Physician Aid In Dying, Making it the Fifth State to Authorize Medical Aid in Dying.

CHAPTER THREE

U.S. Laws On Assisted Death

Federal Laws:

1) There are no specific federal laws regarding euthanasia or assisted death.
2) All fifty states and the District of Columbia prohibit euthanasia under general homicide laws.
3) Assisted death laws are handled at the state rather than the federal level.

State Laws:

1) Thirty-eight states have specific laws prohibiting all assisted deaths.
2) Three states prohibit all assisted deaths under common law.
3) Four states and the District of Columbia have no specific laws regarding assisted death, and do not recognize common law in regard to assisted death.
4) Five states – Oregon, Montana, Washington, Vermont, and New Mexico – have legalized physician-assisted dying.

CHAPTER FOUR

King George V's Drug-Induced Death

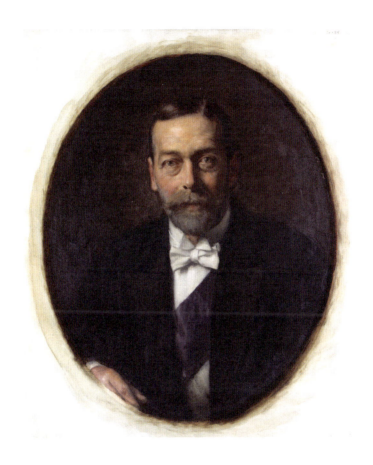

One should make the act of dying more gentle and more peaceful even if it does involve curtailment of the length of life.

Lord Dawson
King George V's Physician

On January 20, 1936, King George V was injected with a lethal dose of morphine and cocaine to hasten his death. His physician, Lord Dawson, administered the injection after consulting with the King's wife and son – they saw no point in prolonging the King's suffering since his condition, cardiorespiratory disease, was terminal. In fact, Lord Dawson agreed with Queen Mary, who told him to not "strive officiously" to keep the King alive. In notes that he made after the King's death, Lord Dawson wrote: "It was evident that the last stage might endure for many hours, unknown to the patient but little comporting with the dignity and the serenity which he so richly merited and which demanded a brief final scene." King George's death via a lethal injection was kept hidden from the public for fifty years.

CHAPTER FIVE

ALS:

Lou Gehrig's Disease

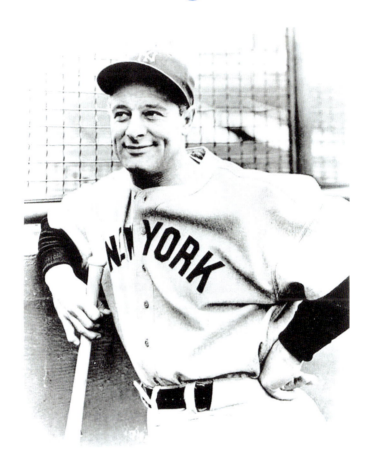

What we have done for ourselves alone dies with us; what we have done for others and the world remains and is immortal.

Albert Pike

Lou Gehrig, the New York Yankee's spectacular first baseman, was nicknamed the Iron Horse because he had played in 2,130 straight games, with 493 home runs, 13 consecutive 100-RBI seasons, and a .340 career average. On July 4, 1939, after several days of news reports about his diagnosis of Amyotrophic Lateral Sclerosis (ALS), Gehrig spoke to a crowd of 62,000 fans at Yankee Stadium. He announced that he had "gotten a bad break," but considered himself "the luckiest man on the face of this Earth." He died less than two years later.

ALS is a terminal disease. It causes a hardening of the spinal cord, which leads to a slow and painful deterioration of muscles and nerve endings, followed by paralysis and eventual heart and lung failure. ALS strikes at random, killing young and old inexorably. The cruelest part of the disease is that the mind is unaffected, and patients are usually fully cognizant and coherent until a few weeks before their death. It is an excruciating demise. In 2014, 75 years after Lou Gehrig's announcement, ALS is just as unbearable, crippling, degrading, and lethal as it was in 1939.

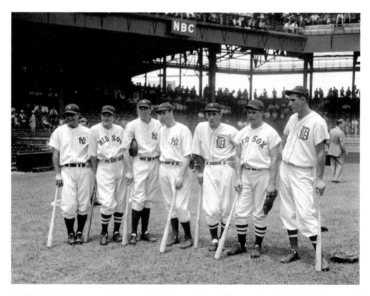

1937 All-Stars: Lou Gehrig, Joe Cronin, Bill Dickey, Joe DiMaggio, Charlie Gehringer, Jimmie Foxx, Hank Greenberg

CHAPTER SIX

Karen Quinlan: The Right To Die

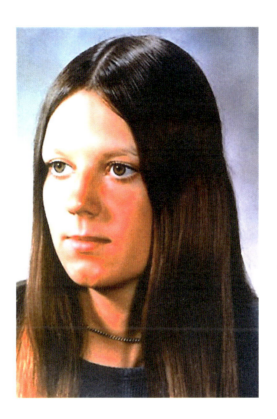

That grey console called the respirator, with its lights blinking on and off like some giant electronic computer, making hissing and gurgling noises as it endlessly pumped air down into a hole in Karen's throat…

Julie Quinlan, asking for the removal of her daughter's respirator.

The Karen Quinlan court case was the first "right to die" lawsuit in U.S. history. The pending issue was determining how far medical technology should be allowed to advance to keep someone alive, when it has been established that brain function and quality of life are irreversibly damaged.

On April 14, 1975, Karen Quinlan, age 21, lapsed into a coma after consuming a combination of alcohol and sedatives. By the time paramedics arrived, she was in a vegetative state due to a lack of oxygen to her brain.

Karen was kept alive with feeding tubes and a respirator. Although doctors determined that she had some low-level brain function, she had lost all cognitive abilities. After several months passed with no improvement in her condition, Karen's parents decided to disconnect the machines that were keeping her alive and let her die peacefully.

However, the state of New Jersey intervened, warning that it would prosecute any doctor who helped to end Karen's life. In a New Jersey Superior court room, the Quinlan's asked for permission to remove their daughter from life support. A court-appointed guardian for Karen argued that her parents were proposing euthanasia, and the Quinlan's lost their first legal battle.

They then took their case to the New Jersey Supreme Court, and it ruled that "No compelling interest of the state could compel Karen to endure the unendurable" – and that removing her from life support did not constitute a homicide since Quinlan's death would ensue from natural causes. Karen was finally removed from the respirator in 1976. She continued to receive artificial nutrition and hydration, and lived another ten years before dying of pneumonia at the age of thirty-one. The autopsy revealed severe damage to her thalamus, the part of the brain that processes sensory information.

The Karen Quinlan lawsuit was a milestone for setting legal precedents:

- **Right-to-Die Cases and Bioethics:** Discussing the moral and ethical issues at the end of life.
- **Medical Treatments:** Establishing a patient's right to refuse medical treatments.

- **Health Care Decisions:** Changing the way health care decisions are made by creating ethics committees in hospitals, nursing homes, and hospices nationwide.

Creation of Advance Directives and Health Care Proxies.

Implicit in the Quinlan verdict was the fact that end-of-life decisions needed to be codified, and that the ethical debate – medical advances prolonging life – would continue to be an unresolved issue.

CHAPTER SEVEN

Terri Schiavo:

Vegetative State

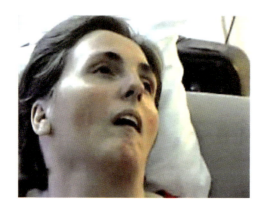

Persistent Vegetative State (PVS)

And then they sign an affidavit swearing that she's not in a vegetative state. I'll tell you. That's a doctor you really want; they can look at a picture and make a diagnosis... They have a list of doctors that signed affidavits from looking at a picture of Terry.

Michael Schiavo
Terri's husband

The Terri Schiavo legal case turned into a campaign to determine how long a patient should be given life support, after the patient has been diagnosed in a vegetative state. Due to activism by pro-life and disability rights movements, the Schiavo lawsuit soon became known throughout the U.S.

On February 25, 1990, Terri Schiavo suffered a full cardiac arrest, resulting in massive brain damage due to a lack of oxygen. After two and a half months in a coma, she was diagnosed in a "persistent vegetative state" – a state of partial arousal caused by severe brain damage.

For the next few years, doctors experimented with speech and physical therapy, with the hope of returning her to a state of awareness. After all attempts failed, Terri's husband, Michael Schiavo, asked for the right to terminate his wife's life support, but Terri's parents and the state of Florida opposed him.

At issue were the uncertainty of Terri's consciousness, and the question of whether Michael Schiavo had the right to turn off her life support, when Terri's parents, Robert and Mary Schindler, opposed it.

In 1998, Michael Schiavo petitioned the Sixth Circuit Court of Florida to remove Terri's feeding tube. The court determined that Terri would not choose to have life-prolonging procedures, and on April 24, 2001, ordered the removal of her life support. There were several appeals and government interventions, including President George W. Bush returning to Washington D.C. to sign legislation intended to keep her alive.

All of the appeals through the federal court system upheld the original decision to remove Terri's feeding tube, and it was finally disconnected on March 18, 2005. Terri died two weeks later, on March 31, 2005.

Litigation in the Schiavo case included: fourteen appeals; numerous motions, petitions, and hearings; five lawsuits in federal district court; and four denials from the U.S. Supreme Court.

CHAPTER EIGHT

Sue Rodriguez:

"Who Owns My Life?"

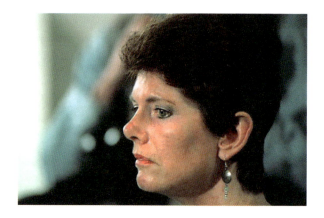

If I cannot give consent to my own death, whose body is this? Who owns my life?

Sue Rodriguez
ALS patient, 1992

In a videotape presented to Members of Parliament and the Supreme Court of Canada, Sue Rodriquez, age forty-one, asked legislators for the "right to die."

Sue was diagnosed with ALS in 1991. Her first symptoms were twitching and tightness in her hands and arms, along with pain in her neck and lower back. Sue's doctor told her that she would eventually lose the ability to walk, talk, and even breathe, and that the average life expectancy after diagnosis was three to five years.

Although counseling and aiding someone to commit suicide is illegal in Canada, committing suicide is not. Sue's attorney argued that the ban on physician-assisted death violated her rights of liberty and autonomy according to the Charter of Rights and Freedoms, and as a consequence, was unconstitutional. In *Rodriguez v. British Columbia* (Attorney General) (1993), Canada's Supreme Court rejected those arguments in a 5-4 ruling, asserting that the state's right to preserve life and protect those who are weak and defenseless outweighed Sue's personal rights.

In 1994, Sue Rodriguez circumvented the courts, and with the aid of an anonymous doctor, she attained the assisted-death that Canada's Supreme Court had denied her.

CHAPTER NINE

Dr. Jack Kevorkian:

Hero Or Criminal?

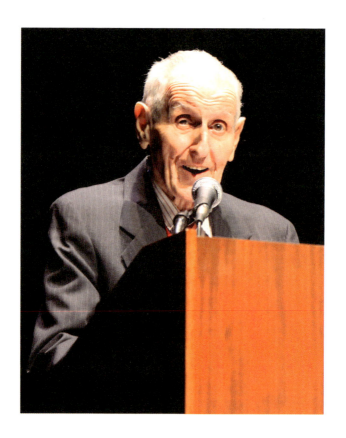

If you don't have liberty and self-determination, you've got nothing, that's what this country is built on. And this is the ultimate self-determination, when you determine how and when you're going to die when you're suffering.

Dr. Jack Kevorkian

On November 22, 1998, the CBS show *60 Minutes* aired Dr. Jack Kevorkian performed voluntary euthanasia on Thomas Youk, age fifty-two. Youk had been suffering from Lou Gehrig's disease, and he had asked Dr. Kevorkian to help end his life. Accordingly, Kevorkian injected him with enough poison to stop his heart. It was riveting television.

Jack Kevorkian was born on May 28, 1928, in Pontiac, Michigan. A graduate of the University of Michigan's medical school, his colleagues dubbed him "Dr. Death" because of his intense interest in dying patients. During the 1980s, Kevorkian worked in hospitals in California and Michigan, and wrote articles on voluntary euthanasia that were published in European medical journals. Kevorkian was living in Holly, Michigan when he built his first "suicide machine" – a mechanism that allowed the operator to self-inject an anesthetic, followed by a lethal dose of potassium chloride. In 1990, Jane Adkins, age fifty-four and suffering from Alzheimer's, asked Kevorkian to assist in terminating her life, and she became Kevorkian's first patient to die in his Volkswagen van "suicide machine."

Kevorkian continued to "assist" patients who were suffering from terminal or incurable illnesses, and the state of Michigan initiated a 1993 law that *explicitly* prohibited him from aiding in any more deaths. He nevertheless defied the decree, forcing the issue of assisted dying into the courts and into mainstream media. As he became more and more famous, appearing on the cover of *Time* magazine, in newspaper columns, and on TV talk shows across the nation, he was both celebrated and reviled.

And so in 1998, when he gave *60 Minutes* the videotape of Thomas Youk's death, his intention was to once again provoke the legal establishment and force the issue of voluntary euthanasia into mainstream deliberations. However, because Kevorkian had lost his medical licenses in California and Michigan, his use of potassium chloride (shown in the videotape) was illegal, and he was charged with the delivery of a controlled substance and second-degree murder. In 1999, Kevorkian was convicted and sentenced to 10-25 years in prison. Due to failing health, he was granted early parole and released from prison in 2007. He lived in the Detroit area until his death in 2011.

Jack Kevorkian devoted his life to changing assisted death laws in Michigan and in the U.S. There is no question that Kevorkian, more than any other individual, brought the issue of physician-assisted death to the forefront of American society. In the final analysis, he helped 130 people who were suffering from intolerable pain to end their lives with dignity, knowing full well that he would lose his dignity by ending up in prison. Jack Kevorkian was a hero for our time.

CHAPTER TEN

Stairway To Heaven:

How To Die In Oregon

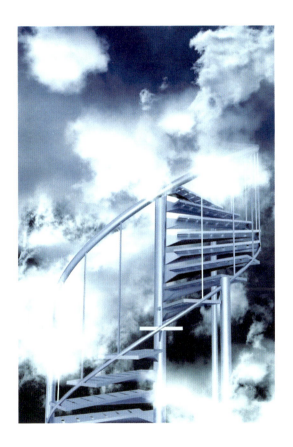

There walks a lady we all know. Who shines white light and wants to show. How everything still turns to gold… And she's buying a stairway to heaven.

Led Zeppelin
Stairway To Heaven

In 1994, the electorate in Oregon voted for "Death With Dignity" legislation, and for the first time in U.S. history, medical aid in dying became legal in an American state. The documentary ***How To Die In Oregon*** is a compassionate portrayal of terminal patients who are overwhelmed by their illnesses, whether it's due to excruciating pain or a life without dignity, or in most cases, both.

How To Die In Oregon (produced by HBO) reveals the nobility behind Death With Dignity laws, since it chronicles men and women with terminal illnesses who have opted for assisted death. Executive Producer/Director Peter Richardson interviewed patients, family members, and health care practitioners, asking the questions that most people would ask, and that's what makes this documentary so powerful: It could be you or me. At least, for most of these patients, there was the option of a "good death." For the majority of Americans, that option does not exist.

One of the stories documented in ***How To Die In Oregon*** portrays the final ten months of one woman's life:

During the winter of 2008-2009, Cody Curtis, age 54, had a recurrence of liver cancer, along with the estimation that she only had six months or less to live. Cody decided to keep a lethal amount of Seconal in her home, in case her life became intolerable. Just having the option of assisted death was an enormous relief for her: The comfort of knowing that she would not have to suffer the indignities and pain she had been forced to endure during her first bout with liver cancer; the knowledge that she didn't have to put her husband and two grown children through the agony of seeing her in excruciating pain again; and knowing that she had an out – gave her peace of mind and security.

Cody outlived her prognosis, possibly because she didn't have chemotherapy or radiation, and therefore, didn't have to suffer the horrific side effects from either of those "treatments." She lived ten months instead of six, and for a few of those months, she felt remarkably well.

Throughout the ten months recorded by Richardson's camera, Cody was hopeful that she would "drift off" in her sleep, rather than having to make the decision to end her life with a lethal amount of a drug. Unfortunately, her illness became too distressing and too painful to live with, and when she finally decided to ingest the Seconal, her family and doctor were by her side.

Cody had almost one year to say "good-bye" to her family and friends – to have a real farewell. And at the end, with her dignity intact, she chose to have a "good and gentle" death.

For everyone living in the U.S., Canada, Britain, and other countries, this is a must-see documentary. *How To Die In Oregon* reveals the empathy and humanity of "Death With Dignity" legislation, and why every terminally ill patient should have the option of assisted death.

CHAPTER ELEVEN

Oregon

Washington

Montana

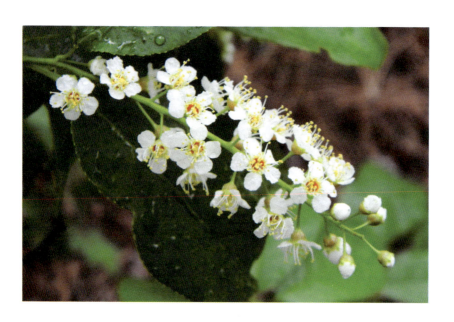

Death With Dignity Laws

"Death With Dignity" laws apply to terminally ill patients who are judged, by physicians, to be mentally competent and capable of making the decision to hasten their death via a lethal dose of a medication. Terminally ill patients in Oregon, Washington, and Montana can choose to accelerate their death by minutes, hours, weeks, or months, due to agonizing pain, lack of quality of life, or both. In all three states, the patient must have a terminal or incurable illness in order to have the legal option of physician aid in dying. The intent of assisted death laws is to curtail suffering and give patients the opportunity to have a peaceful death.

Oregon: Nov. 8, 1994

- **How Passed (Yes Vote):** Ballot Measure Initiative - 16 (51%)
- **Residency Required**: Yes
- **Minimum Age**: 18
- **Number of months until expected death:** 6 or less.
- **Number of requests to physicians:** Two oral (at least 15 days apart).

Washington: Nov. 4, 2009

- **How Passed (Yes Vote):** Initiative 1000 – (58%)
- **Residency Required**: Yes
- **Minimum Age**: 18
- **Number of months until expected death:** 6 or less.
- **Number of requests to physicians:** Two oral (at least 15 days apart) and one written.

Montana: Dec. 31, 2009

- **How Passed (Yes Vote):** Montana Supreme Court in *Baxter v. Montana* (5-4)
- **Residency Required**: Yes
- **Minimum Age**: *
- **Number of months until expected death:** *
- **Number of requests to physicians:** *
  No legal protocol in place.

Oregon

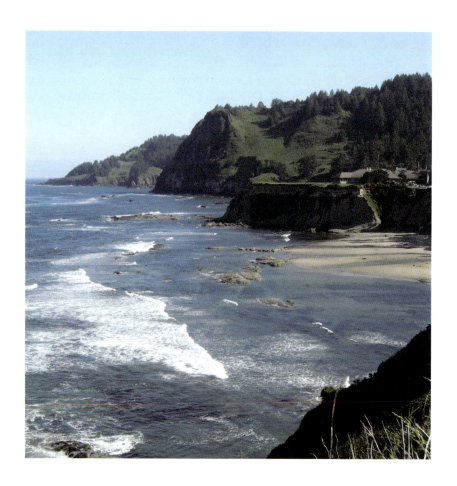

Just as I shall select my ship when I am about to go on a voyage, or my house when I propose to take a residence, so I shall choose my death when I am about to depart from life.

Seneca

Ballot Measure 16: Allows Terminally Ill Adults To Obtain Prescription for Lethal Drugs (Death With Dignity Act)

Decided: Nov. 8, 1994 (51% for)

"An adult who is capable, is a resident of Oregon, and has been determined by the attending physician and consulting physician to be suffering from a terminal disease, and who has voluntarily expressed his or her wish to die, may make a written request for medication for the purpose of ending his or her life in a humane and dignified manner."

Ballot Measure 51: Repeals Law Allowing Terminally Ill Adults To Obtain Lethal Prescription

Decided: Nov. 4, 1997 (60% against)

Supreme Court of the United States: *Gonzales v. State of Oregon*

Decided: Jan. 17, 2006 (6-3 in favor of the State of Oregon)

According to the court's majority opinion, the Controlled Substances Act does not empower the Attorney General of the United States to prohibit doctors from prescribing regulated drugs for use in physician-assisted death under state law permitting the procedure. The court's ruling upheld the Death With Dignity Act.

Oregon Health Authority

Address: 800 Northeast Oregon Street, Portland, OR 97232

Phone #: 971-673-1222

Email: dwda.info@state.or.us

Website: Oregon Health Authority - Death With Dignity Act

- *http://public.health.oregon.gov/ProviderPartnerResources/Eval uationresearch/deathwithdignityact/Pages/index.aspx*

Patient eligibility:

- 18 years of age or older
- Resident of Oregon
- Capable of making and communicating health care decisions for him/herself.
- Diagnosed with a terminal illness that will lead to death within six months.

Physician protocol: The attending physician must be licensed in the same state as the patient.

- The physician's diagnosis must include a terminal illness, with six months or less to live.
- The diagnosis must be certified by a consulting physician, who must also certify that the patient is mentally competent to make and communicate health care decisions.
- If either physician determines that the patient's judgment is impaired, the patient must be referred for a psychological examination.
- The attending physician must inform the patient of alternatives, including palliative care, hospice, and pain management options.
- The attending physician must request that the patient notify their next-of-kin of the prescription request.

Patient request timeline:

- First oral request to physician
- 15 day waiting period
- Second oral request to physician
- Written request to physician
- 48 hour waiting period before picking up prescribed medications.
- Pick up prescribed medications from the pharmacy.

Other:

- Use of the law cannot affect the status of a patient's health or life insurance policies.
- The Department of Human Services - Health Services enforces compliance with the law. Compliance requires physicians to report all prescriptions to the state. Physicians and patients who comply with the law are protected from criminal prosecution.

Physicians and health care systems are not obligated to participate.

Oregon voters passed their "Death with Dignity" act in 1994. Due to many challenges in court, including a challenge and failure by the Supreme Court of the United States, the law did not go into effect until 1997.

Washington

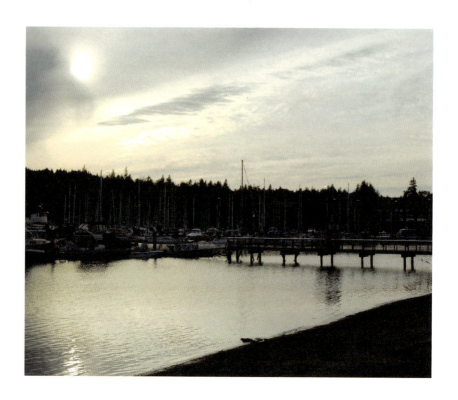

There is no death! What seems so is transition; this life of mortal breath is but a suburb of the life elysian, whose portal we call Death.

Henry W. Longfellow

Ballot Measure 16: Allows Terminally Ill Adults To Obtain Prescription for Lethal Drugs (Death With Dignity Act)

Decided: Nov. 4, 2009 (58% for)

"An adult who is competent, is a resident of Washington state, and has been determined by the attending physician and consulting physician to be suffering from a terminal disease, and who has voluntarily expressed his or her wish to die, may make a written request for medication that the patient may self-administer to end his or her life in a humane and dignified manner..."

Washington State Department of Health

Address: P.O. Box 47856, Olympia, WA 98504-7856

Phone #: 360-236-4030

Email: secretary@doh.wa.gov

Website: Washington State Department of Health - Death With Dignity Act

- *http://www.doh.wa.gov/YouandYourFamily/IllnessandDisease/DeathwithDignityAct.aspx*

Patient eligibility:

- 18 years of age or older
- Resident of Washington
- Capable of making and communicating health care decisions for him/herself.
- Diagnosed with a terminal illness that will lead to death within six months.

Physician protocol:

- The attending physician must be licensed in the same state as the patient.

- The physician's diagnosis must include a terminal illness, with six months or less to live.
- The diagnosis must be certified by a consulting physician, who must also certify that the patient is mentally competent to make and communicate health care decisions.
- If either physician determines that the patient's judgment is impaired, the patient must be referred for a psychological examination.
- The attending physician must inform the patient of alternatives, including palliative care, hospice, and pain management options.
- The attending physician must request that the patient notify their next-of-kin of the prescription request.

Patient request timeline:

- First oral request to physician
- 15 day waiting period
- Second oral request to physician
- Written request to physician
- 48 hour waiting period before picking up prescribed medications.
- Pick up prescribed medications from the pharmacy.

Other:

- Use of the law cannot affect the status of a patient's health or life insurance policies.
- The Department of Health enforces compliance with the law. Compliance requires physicians to report all prescriptions to the state. Physicians and patients who comply with the law are protected from criminal prosecution.
- Physicians and health care systems are not obligated to participate.

State of Washington Department of Health Statistics for 2010:

The vast majority of patients who requested aid in dying were white, well-educated, insured, dying of cancer, and receiving hospice care. Their reasons for requesting assisted death were loss of autonomy (90 percent), inability to engage in activities that made life enjoyable (87 percent), and loss of dignity (64 percent). A lethal amount of prescription drugs were dispensed to 87 people and 51 of them died after ingesting the drugs; 15 died without having ingested the drugs; 6 died without anyone knowing whether they had ingested the drugs; and the status of the remaining 15 people was unknown. The above data confirms that terminally ill patients who have opted for physician aid in dying in the U.S. have done so under their own volition, in order to experience a peaceful and pain-free death.

Montana

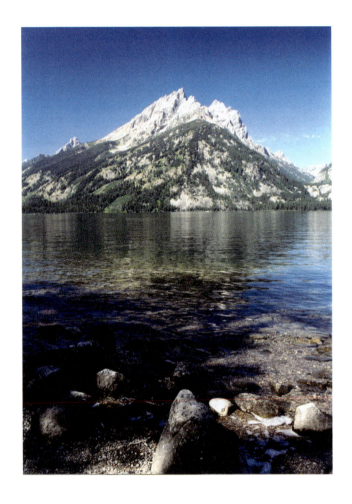

Live as if you were to die tomorrow.
Learn as if you were to live forever.

Mahatma Gandhi

Montana First Judicial District Court: Baxter v. Montana

Decided: Dec. 5, 2008 in favor of plaintiffs

The plaintiffs (four Montana physicians, Compassion and Choices, and Robert Baxter, a 76-year-old truck driver from Billings dying of lymphocytic leukemia) asked the court to establish a constitutional right "to receive and provide aid in dying."

Judge Dorothy McCarter ruled that a terminally ill, competent patient has a legal right to die with dignity under Article II, Sections 4 and 10 of the Montana Constitution. That includes a right to "use the assistance of his physician to obtain a prescription for a lethal dose of medication that the patient may take on his own if and when he decides to terminate his life." It further held that the right protects physicians who aid such patients by prescribing a lethal drug for the patient.

State Supreme Court: *Baxter v. Montana*

Decided: Dec. 31, 2009 in favor of plaintiffs 5-4

The Attorney General of Montana appealed the ruling of Judge McCarter to the Montana Supreme Court. The Court found that "we find no indication in Montana law that physician aid in dying provided to terminally ill, mentally competent adult patients is against public policy" and therefore, the physician who assists is shielded from criminal liability by the patient's consent. On Feb. 17, 2011, the Montana legislature tabled two proposed physician-assisted death bills. According to the Billings Gazette, "one would have banned the practice altogether" (LC0041 - Republican Senator Greg Hinkle), while the other (LC0177 - Democratic Senator Dick Barrett) would have required a doctor to diagnose a patient as being terminally ill and the patient to make voluntary oral and written requests for a lethal prescription of medication. The request would have had to be signed by two witnesses and the patient also would have had to get a second doctor's opinion.

Death With Dignity National Center, on its website at *http://www.deathwithdignity.org*, explains that "existing Montana state law provides immunity for physicians for withholding or withdrawing life-sustaining treatment for a terminally-ill patient," but "does not specifically address physician-assisted death."

(Source: *ProCon.org: http://www.euthanasia.procon.org*)

Safeguards for "Death With Dignity" Laws to Ensure that Patients Cannot be Forced, Intimidated, or Coerced into having Physician Aid in Dying:

Posted by Melissa Barber on April 5, 2011: (Death With Dignity National Center)

(Source*: http://www.deathwithdignity.org/author/melissa-barber*)

- The patient must verbally request the medication from the physician twice, and each request is separated by 15 days.
- In addition, the patient must make a written request to the attending physician, which is witnessed by two individuals who are not primary care givers or family members.
- The patient is notified and is able to rescind the verbal and written requests at any time – even right before the patient ingests the medication.
- The patient must be able to self-administer and ingest the prescribed medication.
- The attending physician must be Oregon or Washington licensed. (No legal protocol in place for Montana.)
- The physician's diagnosis must include terminal illness, with six months or less to live.
- The diagnosis must be certified by a consulting physician, who must also certify the patient is mentally competent to make and communicate health care decisions.
- If either physician determines the patient's judgment is impaired, the patient must be referred for a psychological examination.

- The attending physician must inform the patient of alternatives, including palliative care, hospice, and pain management options.
- The attending physician must request the patient notify their next-of-kin of the prescription request.
- A person who coerces or exerts undue influence on a patient to request medication for the purpose of ending the patient's life shall be guilty of a Class A felony.

Oregon Department of Human Services "Death With Dignity" Statistics - 14 Years:

The Oregon Department of Human Services is required to provide data each year regarding Death With Dignity legislation. Fourteen years of data refutes unsubstantiated predictions by those who oppose aid in dying:

Annual Reports:

- *http://public.health.oregon.gov/ProviderPartnerResources/Eval uationResearch/DeathwithDignityAct/Pages/ar-index.aspx*

Oregon's Law Withstands the Test of Time:

Posted by George Eighmey, Jan. 19, 2011. (Death With Dignity National Center)

(Source: *http://www.deathwithdignity.org/2011/01/19/oregons-law-withstands-test-time*)

- **Myth:** Hundreds of people would use the law each year and hundreds would move to Oregon to use the law.
- **Reality:** In the first year of the law's existence only 16 Oregonians died after completing the process. In 12 years, a total of 460 died using the law; an average of 38 per year. This corresponds to an estimated 19.3 Death With Dignity Act deaths per 10,000 total deaths each year. The law is

seldom used, but it provides comfort to thousands who know it is available if worse becomes worse in their final days.

- **Myth:** Dying people would be coerced into using the law because family members would not want their inheritance depleted. Their slogan was one would have the "Duty to Die."

- **Reality:** In my 12 years facilitating dying Oregonians with the law, not one claimed they were being urged to use the law by their family. In fact, in most cases it was the dying person who had to persuade their loved ones to support them in their decision to use the law. Finally, coercion or exerting undue influence over a patient is a Class A felony under the law, punishable by life in prison and a $50,000 fine.

- **Myth:** 25 percent of the people who consumed the lethal dose of medication would stay alive for more than 3 hours and most of them would awaken to later die an agonizing death.

- **Reality:** The average length of time from consumption of the medication to death is 2 hours with fewer than 4 percent of those who died taking longer than 3 hours. One person out of 460 (1/5 of 1 percent) awakened after taking the medication and the patient later died peacefully.

- **Myth:** Depressed people would abuse the law out of desperation.

- **Reality:** The safeguards in the law require the patient be mentally competent, and if either of two doctors has any concerns about the patient's mental competence, then the patient must be referred for a mental health evaluation.

CHAPTER TWELVE

Netherlands

Belgium

Luxembourg

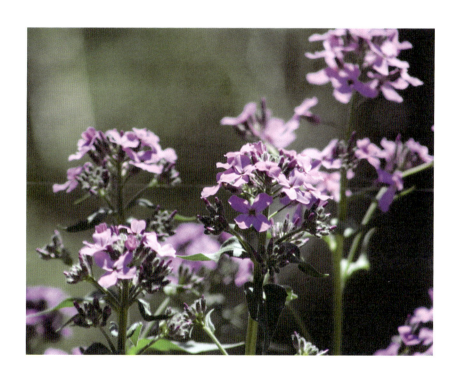

Voluntary Euthanasia Laws

We conclude that the Dutch approach, based on ex ante consultation and ex post review, can be regarded as a responsible way of dealing with the moral and legal issues that surround ending life at a patient's request. A focus on trust, quality guarantees, transparency, and control in the medical profession promotes careful practice, combining patients' rights and interests on the one hand and physicians' integrity and professionalism on the other.

Euthanasia in the Netherlands,
Consultation and Review,
Kings Law Journal,
August 2012

The Netherlands

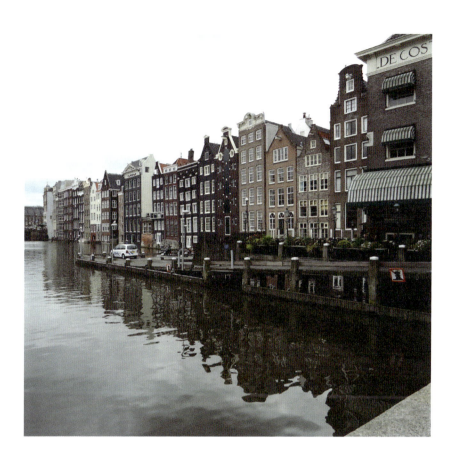

To fear death is nothing other than to think oneself wise when one is not.

Socrates

The Netherlands is usually in the forefront of liberal social movements: In 1984, the Dutch Supreme Court ruled that voluntary euthanasia is legal, provided that physicians follow stringent guidelines. Under Dutch criminal law, doctors could still be prosecuted, so Parliament voted to formally legalize euthanasia in the fall of 2000, making the Netherlands the first nation in the world to sanction assisted death.

The Dutch approach to voluntary euthanasia is to preserve the quality of life, even if that entails death. Rather than prolonging an agonizing and hopeless situation, people can choose a dignified and peaceful transition. The criteria for euthanasia are irreversible and unbearable suffering caused by a fatal or chronic illness.

Dutch Rules for Assisted Death:

1) The patient must be informed about the diagnosis and its prospects.
2) The patient must voluntarily express their unwavering decision to have a doctor end their life, by a medically approved method.
3) A second opinion of an unbiased physician is required, and then the procedure is reviewed by the Board of Prosecutors-General. Physicians and hospitals have the right to decline a euthanasia request, and since the Netherlands is a secular state, religions do not have a vote.

Voluntary Euthanasia is legal under the following conditions:

1) The patient's suffering is unbearable, with no possibility of improvement.
2) The patient's request for euthanasia must be voluntary and continue over time. The request cannot be granted if a patient has a psychological illness, is under the influence of drugs, or under the influence of other people.
3) The patient must be fully aware of their diagnosis, condition, and options. There must be a consultation with at least one other independent doctor, who will confirm the conditions mentioned above.

4) The death must be carried out in a medically appropriate manner, either by the doctor or the patient. A doctor must be present and the patient must be at least 12-years-old, and patients between 12 and 16 years of age require the consent of their parents.

5) The doctor must report the cause of death to the municipal coroner, in accordance with the relevant provisions of the Burial and Cremation Act. A regional review committee assesses whether a case of termination of life on request or assisted death complies with the "Due Care Criteria." Depending on its findings, the case will either be closed, or if the conditions are not met, brought to the attention of the Public Prosecutor.

Dutch laws recognize the validity of a "euthanasia directive" – or a written declaration of will of the patient regarding euthanasia. These declarations can be used when a patient is in a coma or unable to state if they wish to be euthanized under Dutch criminal law.

If a case does not follow the specific conditions of the law, euthanasia is a criminal offense, with the exception of "normal medical practice" situations that are not subject to the restrictions of the law.

In a 2005 study by the *New England Journal of Medicine*, only 0.4 percent of euthanasia cases did not have explicit requests by patients. The Remmelink Report found that 0.8 percent of the deaths at the time were done without an explicit request of the patient. In 59 percent of the cases, the physician had some information about the patient's wish. According to a summary of the report:

"Life was shortened by between some hours and a week at most in 86 percent of the cases. In 83 percent the decision has been discussed with relatives, and in 70 percent with a colleague. In nearly all cases, according to the physician, the patient was suffering unbearably, there was no chance of improvement, and palliative possibilities were exhausted." Voluntary euthanasia is still a relatively uncommon form of death in the Netherlands. In 2010, there were 3,136 cases, a 19 percent increase over 2009, but still only 2.3 percent of all of the 136,058 deaths for that year.

Belgium

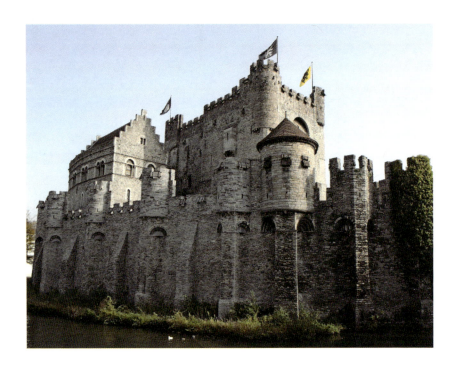

O, let him pass. He hates him. That would upon the rack of this tough world. Stretch him out longer.

King Lear
William Shakespeare

In 2002, voluntary euthanasia was legalized in Belgium under the following conditions: A patient seeking euthanasia must request it more than once; must have a terminal medical condition; and must be continuously suffering, either physically or psychologically.

There were endless hours of discussion, as well as forty Senate hearings, before a euthanasia law was passed, over the objections of the Catholic parties. Those who supported the bill stressed that every citizen should be given the right to choose their last act, according to their private convictions or faith, and that all opinions must be respected. Back in 1997, the Consultative Committee on Bioethics stressed the timeliness of legalizing euthanasia. What changed opinions and perceptions was a comparative analysis of end-of-life decisions between Belgium and the Netherlands that was published in the influential medical journal, the *Lancet*, in 2,000.

The Universities of Brussels, Ghent (Belgium) and Nijmegen (Netherlands) conducted the study: The findings demonstrated that in Belgium – which did not have end-of-life regulations – three quarters of medical decisions to interrupt life were reached without even consulting the patient – the very opposite of what was occurring in the Netherlands.

In another medical study of Belgium, conducted in 2007, the number of cases of voluntary euthanasia increased to nearly two percent of all deaths that year, and there was an increase in all end-of-life decisions, as well. The research group (from the Brussels-based Free University), discovered that the rise was mainly due to Belgium's 2002 euthanasia law, since it gave terminally ill patients more options. In a letter published in the *New England Journal of Medicine*, the group stated:

"We found that the enactment of the Belgian euthanasia law was followed by an increase in all types of medical end-of-life practices, with the exception of the use of lethal drugs without the patient's explicit request."

Dr. Johan Bilsen, who helped conduct the study, said that his team examined a random sample of 6,202 death certificates of people who died between June and November 2007 in Flanders, a Dutch-speaking region, where six million of Belgium's ten million people live. The certifying doctors involved in the study were interviewed, and 118 cases of voluntary euthanasia were found.

Dr. Bilsen discovered a rising trend in assisted death practices from the first Belgian study conducted in 1998. He told the *Associated Press*: "It [euthanasia] has doubled since 1998. It is going up from 1.1 to 1.9 percent."

According to the study, most of the patients who chose euthanasia were younger, had cancer, and died at home. Bilsen noted that the trend reflected similar numbers seen in the Netherlands, after it legalized euthanasia in 2001.

Luxembourg

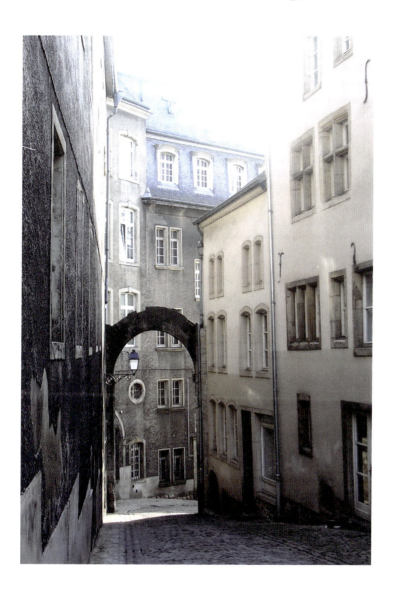

As a well spent day brings happy sleep, so life well used brings happy death.
Leonardo DaVinci

On February 19th 2008, Luxembourg's Parliament voted to legalize voluntary assisted death. The law passed by way of 30 votes to 26. Luxembourg's media called it a "symbolic defeat" for Prime Minister Jean-Claude Junker, who's Christian Social Party opposed it. Euthanasia was approved for the terminally ill, and for those with incurable diseases or conditions, as long as there was the consent of two doctors. On March 18th 2009, Luxembourg enacted the legislation to legalize euthanasia, establishing the nation-state as the third European country to enact assisted death laws.

Jean Huss, a Green Party MP and co-sponsor of the bill, stated that a series of checks and balances were going to be in the bill and that only the terminally ill would be permitted to have assisted death. Socialist lawmaker Lydie Err, who helped draft the bill, avowed: "This bill is not a permit to kill. It's not a law for the parents or the doctors but for the patient and the patient alone to decide if he wants to put an end to his suffering."

People have to repeatedly ask to die, before a witness, and it must be documented, in order for them to receive the consent of two doctors and a panel of experts. In Luxembourg, The Palliative Care and Euthanasia Bill is regulated by a living will or advance directives. Doctors must meet with a colleague to ensure that the patient is either terminally ill or in a "grave and incurable condition." Doctors can then perform assisted death, with a lethal injection or a lethal prescription, without penal sanctions.

As in Belgium, many Catholics opposed voluntary euthanasia in Luxembourg. The Grand Duke of Luxembourg refused to affix his signature to the statute, so Parliament enacted legislation by removing the Grand Duke's veto power. Pope Benedict XVI expressed his "deep concern" for the advancement of euthanasia legislation, insisting that taking innocent human life is always wrong. Jean Huss countered the opposition to euthanasia, by observing: "The Christian Social Party and the Catholic Church were against the euthanasia law, calling it murder but we said no, it's just another way to go."

CHAPTER THIRTEEN

Switzerland:

Tourism Aid In Dying

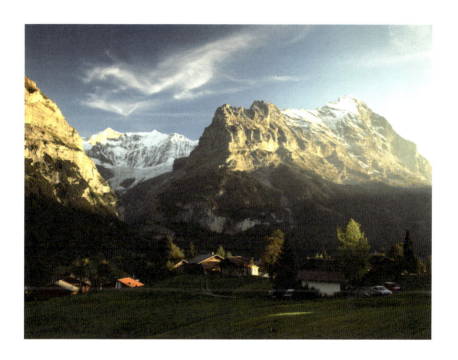

I hate all pain. Given or received, we have enough within us. The meanest vassal as the loftiest monarch, Not to add to each other's natural burden Of mortal misery.

Sardanapalus
LORD BYRON

Assisted death has been legal in Switzerland since 1937. It does not have to be implemented by a physician, and it does not require that a patient be terminally ill. Under Article 115 of the Swiss penal code, assisted death "is a crime if and only if the motive is selfish." Nor does Swiss law consider suicide a crime. Instead, it views suicide as rational.

In Switzerland, it is *motive* that matters, not *intent*. The caveat for assisted death under Swiss law is that people cannot profit from a death. Anyone who assists in a death must do so for purely altruistic reasons. And in contrast to the Netherlands, Belgium, and Luxembourg, physicians do not have a special status.

It is euthanasia that is illegal in Switzerland – a doctor cannot administer a lethal drug to a patient. Swiss law separates the *issue* of whether or not assisted death should be allowed, from that of whether physicians should do it. Instead, patients must take the lethal prescription on their own.

Switzerland is the only country whereby its laws decriminalize assisted death, without requiring the involvement of a physician. Before 2003, assisted death was not even considered to be "part of a physician's activity." During the last decade, doctors have assisted the terminally ill with dying "under strict conditions." An officer from the coroner's department must be in attendance for all assisted deaths, and a doctor can assist under the following circumstances: The death must be videotaped and reported to the police; family and friends must be interviewed; and as long as there isn't a selfish motive, each assisted death is considered an "open-and-shut" case.

In a 1999 survey of the Swiss public, 82 percent of 1000 respondents agreed that "a person suffering from an incurable disease and in intolerable physical or psychological suffering has the right to ask for death and to obtain help for this purpose."

DIGNITAS is a non-physician organization that assists in many of the deaths in Switzerland. Its director, Ludwig Minelli, is a human rights attorney. Exit Switzerland and the Swiss Society for Humane Dying are other organizations that work closely with Switzerland on assisted death.

DIGNITAS has more than 2,000 members and is the only group that welcomes foreigners. Minelli will meet with a foreigner to discuss their death, to make sure that the patient is of sound mind. The foreigner will then meet with a DIGNITAS doctor, who has already reviewed their medical records, and who then prescribes a barbiturate strong enough to kill. The preferred prescription is an overdose of pentobarbital, a sleeping RX. A member of DIGNITAS then takes the foreigner to a rented apartment in Zurich, where the patient then takes the prescription by himself. Patients who are too ill to drink can use a self-induced injection, or a tube through the stomach.

On January 26, 2007, Dr. John Elliott, suffering from multiple myeloma, told Sydney's *Morning Herald* that he was traveling to Switzerland to "die with dignity."

"My name is Dr. John Elliott and I'm about to die, with my head held high…" Three months earlier, a tumor was pressing on his spine and felt like *"a knife in the back and twisting it... Because of my illness I have come to Zurich in Switzerland to use the services of the Dying-With-Dignity organization, DIGNITAS…*

"I have made this trip halfway around the world to try to achieve control of my passing. My disease has dictated that I will soon die and I will die in pain. Worse than this, though, I will have no dignity in death…

"I want to exit this world free and with my head held high… I am not depressed. As one who is medically trained I know depression, and this is not me. I am not even sad. Rather, I have come to Zurich because it is the only legal option available to me as an Australian citizen. I am sharing my story to help our politicians understand why people must be allowed control and responsibility in dying, just like they do in living."

Not everyone is comfortable with the way DIGNITAS operates. Swiss psychiatrist Thomas Schlaepfer, a specialist in depression, supports assisted death, but he does not support DIGNITAS:

"If somebody flies into Zurich Airport, is brought into an interview for an hour and prescribed medication, that's totally wrong," he says.

"That's ethically wrong. Legally, it might be OK in Swiss law, but ethically it's wrong."

Schlaepfer asserts that it is "totally impossible" to find out in a brief visit or two whether someone is of sound mind.

In December of 2008, DIGNITAS received worldwide condemnation because of a Sky documentary that videotaped the assisted death of an American. In 2011, a referendum in the Canton of Zurich was held, to decide whether it should continue to allow foreigners to have assisted death, and seventy-eight percent of the voters agreed to continue the practice.

In Canada, Lee Carter (the plaintiff in *Carter v. Canada* - see Chapter 14) told a court in British Columbia that she and her husband took her 89-year-old mother to Switzerland to use the services of DIGNITAS, spending over $30,000 to end her mother's life.

As long as assisted deaths continue to be illegal in other countries, Switzerland will continue to be the prevailing choice for tourism aid in dying. It's a sad state of affairs that terminally ill patients have to travel to another country to end their lives, instead of being in their own homes and surrounded by loved ones.

CHAPTER FOURTEEN

Gloria Taylor: "Personal Exemption" For Physician-Assisted Death

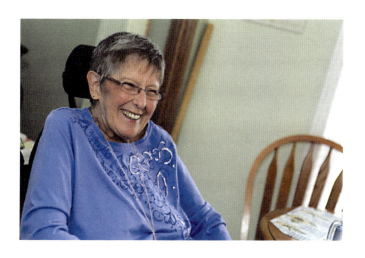

I fear that I will eventually suffocate and die struggling for air like a fish out of water.

After Gloria received a court-ordered "Personal Exemption":

This is a momentous time in history. Now all Canadians will have the "right to die" with dignity. This is a blessing for me and for all other seriously ill Canadians.

In November and December of 2011, attorneys for three sets of plaintiffs and the British Columbia Civil Liberties Association, met in private with attorneys representing the Governments of British Columbia and Canada, to discuss a challenge over physician-assisted death.

Six months later, on June 15, 2012, Madam Justice Lynn Smith of British Columbia's Supreme Court submitted a 395-page decision in *Carter v. Canada*, declaring that Canada's criminal law banning assisted suicide conflicts with the Charter of Rights and Freedoms. As a consequence, she determined that the ban on assisted death is unconstitutional.

Justice Smith granted Gloria Taylor, the main plaintiff in *Carter v. Canada*, and who suffered from Lou Gehrig's disease, a special exemption that accorded her the right to physician-assisted death, at the time of her choosing. For the first time in Canadian history, a citizen was given the "right to die." Justice Smith also instructed the federal government to enact assisted death legislation that did not violate the Charter.

Assisted suicide had been banned, with criminal sanctions, since 1892. Suicide was illegal in Canada, as well, until 1972. For the last forty years, the only prohibition has been against assisted death.

Why was ALS victim, Sue Rodriguez, denied the right to physician-assisted death, when Gloria Taylor, who also suffered from ALS, was given that right two decades later?

When Sue Rodriguez lost her Supreme Court battle in 1993, she was forced to turn to an anonymous physician, who assisted in ending her life in 1994. Since then, the "right to die" movement has gained momentum across North America and Europe: Oregon, Washington, and Montana, and the Netherlands, Belgium, and Luxembourg, enacted assisted death legislation. The scientific data available from assisted-death clinics, worldwide, has demonstrated that there are enough safeguards in place to prevent individuals from being pressured into having assisted dying against their will.

Accordingly, Justice Smith determined that Parliament could create a system of assisted death laws that would have safeguards to protect those who are vulnerable or mentally ill. What had also changed since 1993 were the new interpretive provisions of the Charter by the Supreme Court of Canada: New legal concepts were presented, giving Justice Smith additional laws that she could interpret to assess the constitutionality of the assisted suicide law.

The judge concluded that the law must allow physician-assisted deaths for patients who are diagnosed with a serious illness or disability, and for those who are experiencing "intolerable" physical or psychological suffering, with no chance of improvement. Since the patients in such cases would have to personally request physician-assisted death, and could not be clinically depressed, patients would be free from coercion.

Justice Lynn Smith ruled that the "absolute" prohibition against assisted death is contrary to two rights guaranteed by the *Charter:*

1) The equality guarantee in section 15; and
2) The right to "life, liberty, and security of the person" in section 7. The prohibition is "absolute" because it does not allow for any exceptions, even in limited circumstances.

With this ruling, Madam Justice Smith brought forth into the public arena the debate about assisted death, a discussion that had been closed since *Rodriguez v. British Columbia (Attorney General) 1993*, when the Supreme Court ruled that the assisted suicide provision of the Criminal Code did not breach the Charter. Canada's Attorney General and the Department of Justice had twenty-one days to file a repeal.

Lee Carter and her husband, Hollis Johnson, were plaintiffs in *Carter v. Canada*, as well, since they had facilitated the travel of Lee's 89-year-old mother, Kay, to Switzerland for assisted death. At a news conference, Lee, along with her husband, Hollis, stated that they knew their actions could lead to criminal charges, since it is illegal in Canada to counsel, aid, or abet a person to commit suicide, with the maximum punishment of fourteen years in prison.

Hollis Johnson told reporters: "We definitely knew what we were doing was against the law... I guess sometimes you have to break the law in order to move ahead." Kathleen (Kay) Carter had been diagnosed with spinal stenosis in 2008, while she was living in North

Vancouver. Spinal stenosis disease causes a narrowing of the spine. By 2009, Kay was confined to a wheelchair and unable to dress, feed, or use the bathroom on her own. Her family said that her mind remained sharp, but that she suffered chronic pain and was told by a doctor that she would eventually be lying flat in bed and unable to move.

In July of 2009, Kay asked her daughter and son-in-law to help arrange medical aid in dying. The couple agreed, and did not discuss their plans outside of the family, since they were afraid that Canadian authorities would interfere.

They filled out paperwork that consisted of Kay's medical records and statements that she was of sound mind, and then sent it to DIGNITAS. After medical consultations at the DIGNITAS facility in Zurich, Kay was given a lethal dose of sodium pentobarbital, dissolved in liquid, which she drank using a straw.

Although Kay fell unconscious within minutes, a staff member advised Kay's family that she could still hear them talking, so they reminisced about family memories. Kay was pronounced dead approximately twenty minutes after she ingested the medication. Lee Carter stated that the cost of her mother's assisted death, which included travel expenses, was about $30,000.

Dr. William Shoichet, who lives in Victoria, British Columbia, was the third plaintiff in *Carter v. Canada*, because he volunteered, in the court document, that he would be willing to participate in physician-assisted deaths:

"Dr. Shoichet would require that he be satisfied the patient in question was fully informed, had given due and proper consideration to the issue, and was expressing a continuing and genuine desire for death."

The Court also gave the British Columbia Civil Liberties Association "public interest standing" in *Carter v. Canada*, since it represents patients' rights in health care cases. Grace Pastine, its litigation director, stated that the time was right for the legal challenge, since medical aid in dying was legal in three states in the U.S. and in three countries in Europe. Grace Pastine argued that mentally-competent adults, suffering from serious and incurable illnesses, should have the right to physician-assisted death under certain safeguards, which included multiple doctor's visits and assurances that the person making the choice to end their life was mentally competent. Although the case was filed in British Columbia's Supreme Court, Pastine had the insight to state that *Carter v. Canada* would probably end up in the Supreme Court of Canada.

Carter *v.* Canada FACTS (Court Document):

The three plaintiffs in Carter v. Canada, challenged section 241(b), of the Canadian Criminal Code:

Counseling or aiding suicide

241. Everyone who

- (*b*) aids or abets a person to commit suicide, whether suicide ensues or not, is guilty of an indictable offence and liable to imprisonment for a term not exceeding fourteen years.

Plaintiffs in Carter:

1) Gloria Taylor, who suffers from a fatal, neurodegenerative disease called amyotrophic lateral sclerosis (also known as "ALS");
2) Lee Carter and her husband Hollis Johnson, who helped Ms. Carter's mother to arrange an assisted death in Switzerland, knowing that providing this assistance could expose them to criminal charges in Canada;
3) Dr. William Shoichet, a BC-based family doctor who would be willing to participate in physician-assisted dying if it were no longer illegal and he was convinced that it was appropriate medical care in the circumstances.

The British Columbia Civil Liberties Association was also granted public interest standing in the case as it has a "long-standing interest in matters of patients' rights and health policy" and has some involvement in advocacy regarding end-of-life policy.

The case mainly centered on the first plaintiff, Gloria Taylor. As an ALS patient, Ms. Taylor will lose her physical capacity over time, while retaining all cognitive and mental faculties. While she is currently able to live fairly independently, Ms. Taylor wants to know that she can have a physician-assisted death when she is no longer able to move physically and her life becomes unbearable to her. As she stated in her affidavit before the Court:

"My present quality of life is impaired by the fact that I am unable to say for certain that I will have the right to ask for physician-assisted dying when that 'enough is enough' moment arrives... As Sue Rodriguez asked before me – whose life is it anyway?"

The day the Court's verdict was announced, in June of 2012, Gloria Taylor told reporters that she could not wash herself unaided or perform basic household tasks. She proclaimed that her disease was *"an assault not only on my privacy, but on my dignity and self-esteem."* Gloria frequently had to use a respirator: *"I fear that I will eventually suffocate and die struggling for air like a fish out of water."*

Gloria's lead attorney, Civil Liberties defender Joseph Arvay, told the court that assisted deaths were taking place despite the ban, which he compared to illegal "back-alley abortions" of a few decades ago.

The *Canadian Medical Association Journal* published an editorial calling for a nation-wide debate, insisting that the fate of the assisted-death laws should be decided through the democratic process in voting initiatives, rather than Parliament or in the courts.

The Royal Society of Canada (RSC), the country's senior scholarly body, had stated in a report issued on November 15th 2011, that assisted death in Canada should be regulated and monitored, rather than criminalized. The report coincided just a day after the commencement of *Carter v. Canada*. Its panel of professors and specialists in medical ethics and health law wrote: "A significant majority of the Canadian population appears to support a more permissive legislative framework for euthanasia and assisted suicide."

The RSC report stated that legalizing voluntary euthanasia does not "result in vulnerable persons being subject to abuse or a slippery slope from voluntary to non-voluntary euthanasia. The evidence does not support claims that decriminalization will have a corrosive effect on access to or the development of palliative care."

The RSC maintained that the report was "designed to be balanced, thorough, independent, free from conflict of interest, and based on a deep knowledge of all of the published research that is pertinent to the questions that have been posed."

Canadian Federal Government Launches Appeal:

Carter v Canada (Attorney General) (2012): BC Court Rules that Ban on Assisted Suicide is Unconstitutional

August 7, 2012

Author: Leah McDaniel

In August of 2012, following Justice Smith's verdict, Canada's Conservative federal government launched an appeal of both the declaration of invalidity of the law and the exemption for Gloria Taylor. The government's legal argument was filed with British Columbia's Court of Appeal. Ottawa claimed that legalizing physician-assisted dying would demean the value of life and could hurt people who are vulnerable.

In its 54-page legal argument, the government stressed that people with disabilities, the elderly, and the terminally ill, could be coerced to end their lives, in moments of depression and despair, and that the purpose of the current laws were to protect the vulnerable: "It is a reflection of the state's policy that the inherent value of all human life should not be depreciated by allowing one person to take another's life."

Canada's federal government argued that the Supreme Court's ruling in the Rodriguez case was final, and that British Columbia's

Supreme Court does not have the right to attempt to overrule that decision. In the twenty years since the Rodriguez case, Parliament had examined the assisted death issue several times, and Members of Parliament (MP's) opted to keep the status quo, rather than legalize physician-assisted death, since they feared that there were too many inherent risks associated with voluntary euthanasia. In recent years, Parliament had dealt with nine private MP's bills on this issue: three had failed to gain any support; and six were debated in the House and voted down.

The federal government also claimed that it was Parliament's responsibility to decide whether to authorize euthanasia legislation, and not the court's, which contradicted their argument that Canada's Supreme Court ruling in the Rodriguez case was final.

Department of Justice Attorney Donna Nygard maintained that the government regards life as so sacrosanct that euthanasia or physician-assisted deaths can never be justified. As such, the federal government opposed a constitutional challenge to a Criminal Code sanction that would make physician-assisted death legal in Canada: "Where the state draws the line is that we will not condone the taking of life."

Judge Smith referred Ms. Nygard to a 1972 decision by Parliament to repeal a law that made attempting suicide illegal, saying "the effect was to leave it to the discretion of an individual, rather than to criminalize an attempt to take one's own life."

Ms. Nygard replied that Parliament's aim was not to condone suicide: Instead, they wanted to shift the focus to finding non-legal solutions to preventing suicide.

"The fact is the state stepped back… thus leaving a space of liberty for people to attempt that act," Judge Smith stated.

"The intent was not at all to provide people with the opportunity to commit suicide… [It was] a recognition there was no prohibitive effect [to the law]," Ms. Nygard replied.

Nygard continued to argue that decriminalizing euthanasia and physician-assisted death could lead to the accidental taking of life, such as in cases of critically ill patients unable to communicate their wishes. Ms. Nygard dismissed the fact that a living will would prevent such mistakes from occurring.

Judge Smith reminded everyone that [the state] sends young men and young women off to war, and that the state therefore participated in the deaths of its citizens. Ms. Nygard claimed that war is a "separate and different issue" that isn't relevant to the case, adding: "The exceptional nature of war is such that criminal law doesn't apply… There is a completely different set of rules."

She also claimed there is a difference between the state "condoning" or approving the taking of a life, and "excusing" the taking of life, such as it does when a person kills someone in self-defense. Ms. Nygard further argued that euthanasia or assisted suicide for the terminally ill could not be legalized because that would run counter to basic societal values and the will of Parliament:

"Right now in our society, we do not condone the taking of life… but the legalization of assisted suicide and euthanasia would condone that, and that's where we say there would be a fundamental shift in societal values."

Ms. Nygard also noted that the Supreme Court looked at the issue nine years ago, when it rejected an application from a man dying of AIDS, who asked for an exemption to the law so that he could have physician-assisted death. According to Nygard, the Supreme Court's rejection of that application reinforced its 1993 ruling against Sue Rodriguez. Finally, she claimed that there was no reason to think Canada's Supreme Court would view this issue differently than it had in the past.

Dr. Will Johnston, of the Euthanasia Prevention Coalition of Canada (EPC), agreed with the federal government, warning that people would be forced into assisted death, and called the RSC report "a euthanasia manifesto disguised as an impartial report."

The EPC, which had called the Royal Society of Canada's report urging legalization of euthanasia a "sham," supported and welcomed the news of the appeal in the Carter case. EPC executive director, Alex Schadenberg, wrote on his blog:

"EPC is pleased that Justice Minister Nicholson appealed the disturbing decision by Justice Smith. Minister Nicholson has also appealed the 'constitutional exemption' that was given to Gloria Taylor that he referred to as a 'regulatory framework for assisted suicide.' The decision by Justice Smith needs to be overturned because legalizing euthanasia or assisted suicide is simply not safe."

Schadenberg warned that his organization would intervene in the court case. He maintained that safeguards would not work and that the key is to provide a proper level of care so that patients would not feel that they were living without dignity.

The issue of assisted death in Canada in 2012 could not have been more animated and impassioned for people on both sides of the issue.

On August 11, 2012, Justice Jo-Ann Prowse upheld Gloria Taylor's "right to die." Justice Prowse ruled that reversing Taylor's exemption, the only case of physician aid in dying in Canada's history, would cause her irreparable harm, beyond the interests of the federal government and the public:

"I accept that the exemption has important symbolic and, perhaps, psychological value, which extends beyond Ms. Taylor to those who are similarly situated, whether or not they agree with the decision under appeal," Justice Jo-Ann Prowse wrote in her decision. "She may be a symbol, but she is also a person… and I do not find that it is necessary for the individual to be sacrificed to a concept of the 'greater good,' which may, or may not, be fully informed."

Justice JoAnn Prowse also observed that Gloria might not survive to see the end of her case, as it seemed destined to go to the Supreme Court of Canada. If the exemption were removed and Gloria's health continued to decline, "all of her worst fears would be realized and she would be forced to endure the very death which she has fought so assiduously to avoid," wrote Prowse.

Gloria's attorney, Sheila Tucker, proclaimed:

"She [Gloria] will be delighted with the decision. We're particularly pleased with the fact that the court was very cognizant of the fact that, for Gloria, it really is a case of irreparable harm, because she'll either get to use that exemption and have the value of that exemption now, or she never will… We're very pleased that the court recognized how important it is to Gloria, and how from her perspective it's a right."

At this point, Gloria had not made a decision or taken any formal steps to use her physician-assisted death exemption. In June 2012, after she was granted the right to assisted death, Gloria had announced: *"This is a momentous time in history. Now all Canadians will have the "right to die" with dignity. This is a blessing for me and for all other seriously ill Canadians."*

On October 2, 2012, Gloria Taylor died unexpectedly, from a severe infection caused by a perforated colon. Gloria passed away in a hospital, surrounded by her family and friends.

The British Columbia Civil Liberties Association (BCCLA) released this statement: "Due to the acute nature and brief course of her illness from the infection, Gloria did not need to seek the assistance of a physician to end her life… In the end, Gloria's death was quick and peaceful."

Gloria's mother, Anne Fomenoff, told the press: "We are grateful that Gloria was given the solace of knowing that she had a choice about how and when she would die. Thanks to the ruling of the B.C. Supreme Court, Gloria was able to live her final days free from the fear that she would be sentenced to suffer cruelly in a failing body… I am so proud of my feisty, determined daughter – she struggled to make the world better for Canadians. I speak on behalf of my entire family when I say we are so proud of her legacy. We are blessed to have known and loved this special woman."

The B.C. Supreme Court decision was suspended for one year to give Parliament time to amend the law, and the Appeals Court extended that suspension until after Parliament rendered its decision. The appeal of the declaration of invalidity by B.C. Supreme Court Madam Justice Lynn Smith began in March 2013, and the ruling was overturned at the provincial court level. However, the Supreme Court of Canada is reviewing *Carter v. Canada*, and is expected to have a ruling sometime in 2014. If approved, Canada will become the fifth country to permit medical aid in dying.

Meanwhile, at its February 2014 national convention, Canada's Liberal Party voted to decriminalize aid in dying. Yet, it is the province of Quebec that could pave the way for the rest of the country: The Parti Quebecois introduced Bill 52, which would permit physician aid in dying if the Parti Quebecois wins the April 7th 2014 election. Quebec could potentially pass the most comprehensive end-of-life legislation in North America.

CHAPTER FIFTEEN

Tony Nicklinson:

The Trapped Man

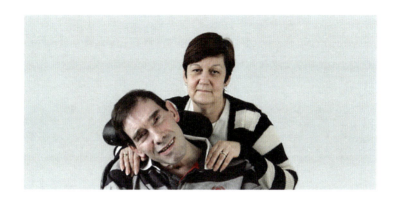

I'm already dead – don't mourn for me.

Tony Nicklinson

When he shall die, Take him and cut him out in little stars. And he will make the face of heaven so fine, That all the world will be in love with night. And pay no worship to the garish sun.

William Shakespeare

In 2005, Tony Nicklinson suffered a catastrophic stroke that left him with "locked-in syndrome." Although his intellect remained intact, he was paralyzed from the neck down, trapped inside his own body.

Prior to his stroke, Tony had enjoyed a full life, working as an engineer in Hong Kong and Dubai, playing rugby, skydiving, and spending time with his wife and daughters.

Gezz Higgins, a friend and former rugby club teammate, described Tony as a "happy-go-lucky" man: "He was an exceptionally good and sociable guy – the sort of fella who, when he walked into a room, you knew things would liven up a bit."

BBC Journalist Lee Stone, who knew Nicklinson before his stroke, was stunned to see a slumped, "twisted and broken" man in a wheel chair.

When Stone attempted to talk to Tony, he could only answer by blinking letters to his wife, Jane. As she tried to interpret what he was saying, Tony drooled and coughed incessantly and Stone began to comprehend what it was like to be "locked-in." Tony had decided to campaign for the "right to die" via Britain's court system, and he shared his opinions and legal documents with Stone, who observed, "His life was the stuff of nightmares."

Since the only way Tony could communicate was by blinking, he used a Windows software program with two cameras that tracked his eye movement, thus enabling him to operate a computer. His goal was to amend Britain's suicide and murder laws in order to end his own life, a life that was intolerable, humiliating, and more painful than most people could ever appreciate.

Nicklinson presented his case for doctor-assisted death to Britain's High Court:

"I have locked-in syndrome and it makes my life a living nightmare. I cannot speak and I am also paralyzed below the neck, which means I need someone to do everything for me. What I find impossible to live with is the knowledge that, unlike you, I have no way out – suicide -- when this life gets too much to bear.

For example, ninety percent of itches have to be endured because by the time someone comes to scratch it and I have laboriously explained where it is, the itch has gone. Now I just put up with them.

Or there is the screaming frustration of wanting to make a point but knowing that the only way I can express my opinion, by the board or computer, are useless in normal conversation.

Another example is having your teeth cleaned by someone else. It is a horrible experience and I doubt you would want it done more than once a day. I could go on. However, all these things are physical and arguably one can learn to live with them.

Assisted dying is a controversial issue which aims to help people to die who are physically unable to take their own life or who can take their own life but want help to do so.

I must declare an interest because I am unable to take my own life. I require amendment to the murder law to make it lawful in certain circumstances for one person to take another's life (euthanasia) and [this] is the substance of my imminent court hearing.

Despite moments of gloom at the enormity of my task, I am kept going by the fundamental injustice of my circumstances and the need for change so that others won't have to endure such indignities if they don't want to. We are all individuals and each person deserves an individual solution to his particular circumstances. A one-size-fits-all solution of better care and more of it, such as opponents advocate, is clearly not the answer. The option of assisted dying should be available.

It is astonishing that in 1969 we could put a man on the Moon yet in 2012 we still cannot devise adequate rules governing assisted dying.

Many opponents of assisted dying object because they think it is wrong to take your own or another's life. Recently I asked such people if there was anything I could say to make them change their mind. They both replied there wasn't. I even suggested to one some safeguards for his approval or otherwise. He totally ignored the question. Clearly any discussion with them is a complete waste of time.

Much has been said about the part care plays in assisted dying and the argument is essentially that better care and more of it will expunge all thoughts of taking one's own life.

For most people the debate is often remote from ordinary lives but for me, the debate on assisted dying is truly a matter of (an unhappy) life and (a pain-free) death. The next stroke could affect you or a loved one; would you be happy to end up like me?

I do not say these things to get your sympathy but to get justice. It cannot be acceptable in 21st Century Britain that I am denied the right to take my own life just because I am physically handicapped."

The day of the High Court's decision, Lee Stone and other journalists gathered at Tony's house to hear the verdict: "He burst into tears. He wept like a child, uncontrollably and without dignity. He wept in the way most of us would weep if we were told we were going to die. For Tony, the news was worse. He was going to live."

Three High Court judges, Lord Justice Toulson, Mr. Justice Royce, and Mrs. Justice Macur, unanimously agreed that the court should stick to its long-established legal position, that euthanasia is murder, "however understandable the motives may be." The judges referred to the "terrible predicament" that Nicklinson was in as "deeply moving and tragic," but they determined that end-of-life issues should be decided by Parliament, and warned that physicians and solicitors who encouraged or assisted in the death of another person were "at real risk of prosecution." Assisted death carries a sentence of up to fourteen years of imprisonment in Britain.

Tony Nicklinson required the "right to die" because he was unable to take his own life, and therefore, needed a lethal injection of drugs. Tony's wife, Jane, revealed that Tony was "devastated" by the decision:

"He said that he was heartbroken by the High Court decision that he could not end his life at a time of his choosing with the help of a new doctor. He could not understand how the legal argument on his behalf could not succeed."

Tony observed:

"I suppose it was wrong of me to invest so much hope and expectation into the judgment but I really believed in the veracity of the argument and quite simply could not understand how anybody could disagree with the logic… I guess I forgot the emotional component."

Jane, who is a nurse, described Tony as being "crestfallen, totally devastated, and very frightened," and that he feared for the future and the misery it was bound to bring:

"His posture had become very bad. He was finding it more and more difficult to use his computer because he was so hunched over – and using his computer was about the only thing he had any pleasure with."

"He was in more discomfort than pain – mental pain, yes. He'd never taken painkillers because he said he wasn't in pain but he'd just started to take them and it would take an awful lot for Tony to take painkillers… It was the day after [the High Court decision] that he said to me that the fight had just gone. He said he couldn't take it anymore."

After Tony received the draft judgment on August 12, 2012, he refused food and liquids, contracted pneumonia, and died ten days later, on August 22nd. Jane described the last forty-eight hours of his life as very unpleasant, "but thankfully it was quick. It's just a shame that he couldn't die the way he wanted to die."

Recent polls in Britain demonstrate that about seventy percent of the public believes there should be a change in the laws regarding assisted death. Tony had described his existence as "pure torture" and that he was condemned to live in a state of "suffering and indignity." Jane and their daughters are determined to continue Tony's fight.

Soon after his death, Anna Soubry, Britain's newly appointed Health Minister, recognized that Britain's laws on assisted death needed to be changed: "I think it's ridiculous and appalling that people have to go abroad to end their life instead of being able to end their life at home."

Tony had told his wife and children:

"I'm already dead - don't mourn for me."

Jane observed: "I think in some respects, seven years ago was harder than this because we did lose the old Tony... Nobody should have to suffer like Tony did."

CHAPTER SIXTEEN

Massachusetts – 2012

Physician Aid in Dying Ballot Fails

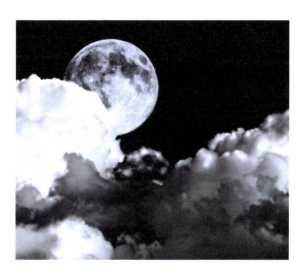

All our knowledge merely helps us to die a more painful death than animals that know nothing.

Maurice Maeterlinck

On November 6, 2012, Massachusetts's voters rejected a "Death With Dignity" ballot measure by a vote of 51 to 49 percent. The question on the ballot stated:

"Should a doctor be legally allowed to prescribe medication, at a terminally ill patient's request, to end that patient's life?"

Ballot approval would have given patients with terminal illnesses and less than six months of life expectancy the opportunity to choose assisted death. Groups that campaigned against the "Death With Dignity" ballot included: disability rights organizations; doctors, nurses, and community leaders; faith-based groups; and patients' rights advocates.

CHAPTER SEVENTEEN

To Gently Leave This Life

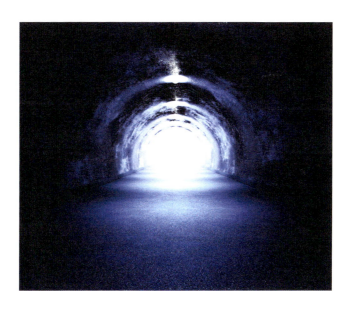

Death - the last sleep? No, it is the final awakening.

Walter Scott

I'm ready to meet my Maker. Whether my Maker is prepared for the great ordeal of meeting me is another matter.

Winston Churchill

In a democracy, the role of government is to allow the individual to live and die according to one's personal convictions, rather than dictate one philosophy over another. At the center of the assisted death debate are the principles of autonomy and free will. Intrinsically, individual end-of-life decisions prevail over government regulations or decrees.

The argument for or against aid in dying typically highlights the ethical deliberation – that assisted death is either right or wrong – when it is, fundamentally, an act of compassion. Medications do not necessarily curtail debilitating pain, and the paradox of state-of-the-art medicine is that it often prolongs life while diminishing one's quality of life and sense of dignity. Moreover, those who argue against life-ending medication deliberately overlook the fact that it is the patient who requests the prescription.

In Ancient Greece and Rome, it was the physician's responsibility to alleviate intolerable suffering by providing a merciful death. Yet in the 21st Century, we force people to suffer until their very last breath. Those who oppose assisted dying can live as long as modern medicine enables them to, but they do not have the moral authority to make end-of-life decisions for others.

In the states that have Death With Dignity laws, most of the people who chose it were college-educated, insured, receiving hospice care, and dying from terminal cancer or another incurable disease. In a 2012 Belgium survey, most of the people who chose voluntary euthanasia were younger, male, had cancer, and chose assisted death due to intolerable pain.

Death With Dignity laws protect the principles of liberty and self-determination pertaining to physicians: If a physician does not want to implement aid in dying, he can refuse and transfer the patient's medical records to another doctor, of the patient's choosing. There is no evidence that assisted death laws have been abused, or that people have been euthanized against their will. The criminalization of assisted dying prevents patients from choosing their own deaths, and prevents physicians from ending their suffering. In contrast, having the "right to die" gives patients the comfort of knowing that they are in control of their lives, if life becomes unbearable, rather than living in fear of a long, agonizing, and undignified death.

It cannot be a coincident that in a 2013 Gallup Poll, seventy-one percent of Americans approved of medical aid in dying, and in a similar British survey, seventy percent of their population supported assisted death as well. Barbara Coombs Lee, president of Compassion and Choices, acknowledged: "People should get the best care, but also have a choice to accelerate the time of death if the very best care cannot make their remaining days acceptable."

In 2014, five states and four countries sanction medical aid in dying. Vermont and New Mexico have jumped on the bandwagon, while Quebec trails closely and deliberately. It is only a matter of time before additional states and countries authorize assisted death legislation. The fact that terminally ill patients, living in states and countries that prohibit assisted dying, have to endure a long and excruciating demise – is poignant and cruel. Whether it is active, passive, voluntary, or involuntary, the option of assisted dying alleviates suffering by offering a peaceful transition.

EPILOGUE

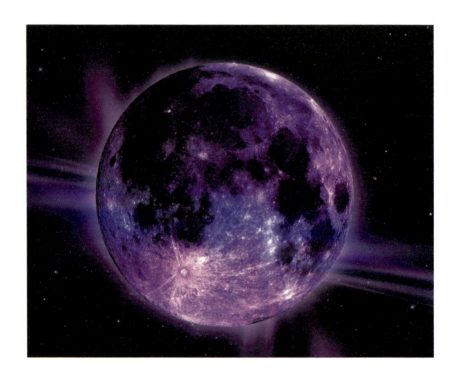

Thank Heaven! The crisis/the danger is past, and the lingering illness is over at last, and the fever called "Living" is conquered at last.

Edgar Allan Poe

In the 21st Century, state-of-the-art medical technology prolongs life as never before. Yet for some people, the issue of greater consequence is the option of a peaceful passing, even if it curtails length of life. Whether it's cutting-edge medical treatments – or medical aid in dying – *man is determining the outcome.*

ALS is one of the most excruciating diseases imaginable. Lou Gehrig died less than two years after he was diagnosed with it, and five decades later, Sue Rodriguez ended her life because of it. In 1998, Dr. Kevorkian assisted an ALS patient with a lethal injection on network TV, and in 2012, a judge in Vancouver granted Gloria Taylor a "personal exemption" for assisted death. However, in Britain, "locked-in" patient Tony Nicklinson pleaded his case to Britain's High Court but was denied the "right to die" despite the tortured nightmare that was his existence.

Whether it's hours, days, weeks, or months, people should have the right to a peaceful transition. Death freely chosen, when we are still cognizant, with our dignity intact, is the gentle and happy passing that has been longed for since the beginning of time.

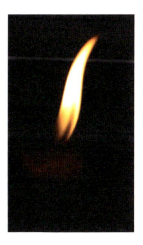

"And all our yesterdays have lighted fools the way to dusty death. Out, out, brief candle! Life's but a walking shadow…"

Macbeth
William Shakespeare

REFERENCES

CHAPTER ONE
Euthanasia: Early Definitions

Dowbiggin, Ian. *A Concise History of Euthanasia: Life, Death, God, and Medicine.* Rowman and Littlefield Publishers, Inc., 2005.

Hurley, D. *Roman Emperors,* 26 April 2004.
http://www.deathwithdignity.org/2011/01/19/oregons-law-withstands-test-time

CHAPTER TWO

History Of Euthanasia

Dowbiggin, Ian. "A Merciful End: The Euthanasia Movement in Modern America," *New England Journal of Medicine,* 4 December 2003. *http://www.deathwithdignity.org/2011/01/19/oregons-law-withstands-test-time*

Emanuel, Ezekiel J., MD. PhD. "The History of Euthanasia Debates in the United States and Britain," *Annals of Internal Medicine,* 15 November 1994. *http://annals.org/article.aspx?articleid=708195*

Emanuel, Ezekiel J., MD. PhD. "Whose Right to Die?" *Atlantic,* March 1997. *http://www.theatlantic.com/magazine/archive/1997/03/whose-right-to-die/304641/*

Manning, Michael, MD. *Euthanasia and Physician-Assisted Suicide: Killing or Caring?* Paulist Press, 1998.
http://books.google.com/books?hl=en&lr=&id=t1THVkQPbfsC&oi=fnd&pg=PR7&dq=Euthanasia+and+Physician-Assisted+Suicide:+Killing+or+Caring%3F&ots=-2PPbgCpDV&sig=OrSvZ6FdBwTyMTxU1rnv3LT579E#v=onepage&q=Euthanasia%20and%20Physician-Assisted%20Suicide%3A%20Killing%20or%20Caring%3F&f=false

Manning, Michael, MD. "Historical Timeline - Euthanasia."
http://euthanasia.procon.org/view.timeline.php?timelineID=000022

"Potter and Euthanasia," *Time,* 31 January 1938.
http://euthanasia.procon.org/view.source.php?sourceID=5192

Ramsay, J.H.R. "A King, a Doctor, and a Convenient Death," *British Medical Journal* (May 1994) 308: 1445.
http://www.bmj.com/content/308/6941/1445.1

Stone, T. Howard; Winslade, William J. "Physician-Assisted Suicide and Euthanasia in the United States," *Journal of Legal Medicine,* December 1995.

CHAPTER THREE

U.S. Laws On Assisted Death

U.S. State and Federal Laws on Euthanasia and Doctor-Assisted Death: http://euthanasia.procon.org/view.resource.php?resourceID=000132

CHAPTER FOUR

King George V's Drug-Induced Death

"A King, a Doctor, and a Convenient Death." J.H.R. Ramsay, *British Medical Journal* (May 1994) 308: 1445.
http://www.bmj.com/content/308/6941/1445.1

Best, Nicholas. *The Kings and Queens of England.* London: Weidenfeld & Nicolson, 1995.
http://books.google.com/books/about/The_Kings_and_Queens_of_England.html?id=fIaoGw AACAAJ

Duke, Barry. Posted in "Assisted Suicide, Euthanasia, Gay, Human Rights," *Free Thinker*, 3 September 2009.
http://freethinker.co.uk/2009/09/03/if-euthanasia-was-good-enough-for-king-george-v-why-should-we-be-denied-it/

Lelyveld, Joseph. "1936 Secret is Out: Doctor Sped George V's Death," *New York Times,* 28 November 1986.
http://www.nytimes.com/1986/11/28/world/1936-secret-is-out-doctor-sped-george-v-s-death.html

CHAPTER FIVE

ALS: Lou Gehrig's Disease

ALS Disease - Lou Gehrig: The Official Web Site.
http://www.lougehrig.com/about/als.html

Amyotrophic Lateral Sclerosis (ALS) - Topic Overview, *WebMD,* 28 January 2011.

"Nutrient CoQ10 May Be an Important Weapon in the Fight Against Lou Gehrig's Disease and Other Neurodegenerative Diseases, Says Anti-aging Institute of California," 18 January 2013.
http://www.b4uage.com/pages/nutrient_coq10_may_be_important_weapon.html

What is ALS? The ALS Association. *http://www.alsa.org/about-als/what-is-als.html*

CHAPTER SIX

Karen Quinlan: The Right To Die

Battelle, Phyllis; Quinlan, Joseph and Julia. *Karen Ann, The Quinlans Tell Their Story.* Bantam Books, 1977.

 "Karen Quinlan Dies, but the Issue Lives On," Posted 11 June 2008.
http://www.wired.com/science/discoveries/news/2008/06/dayintech_0611

Karen Quinlan Photo: Before Coma – 1972.

Long, Tony. "Hypnoxic Brain Injury – What is it?" *Brain Injury Online,* 16 September 2012. *http://www.brain-injury-online.com/hypoxic-brain-injury.html*

Supreme Court Rules in Quinlan Case that Respirator Can Be Removed from Coma Patient, 1976. *http://law.jrank.org/pages/9617/Quinlan-in-Re.html*

CHAPTER SEVEN

Terri Schiavo: Vegetative State

"Compromise Bill Re: Terri Schiavo Signed Into Law: Judge Rules No Re-Insertion of Feeding Tube," *FindLaw,* 20 March 2005.
http://www.findlaw.com

Hentoff, Nat. "Terri Schiavo: Judicial Murder," *Village Voice News,* 22 March 2005.

Terri Schiavo Photo: In Persistent Vegetative State (PVS)

The Terri Schiavo case involved:

14 appeals and numerous motions, petitions, and hearings in the Florida courts; five suits in federal district court; Florida legislation struck down by the Supreme Court of Florida; federal legislation (the Palm Sunday Compromise); and four denials of certiorari from the Supreme Court of the United States. The case also spurred highly visible activism from the pro-life movement and disability rights groups. The Terri Schiavo Life & Hope Network: http://www.terrisfight.org

CHAPTER EIGHT

Sue Rodriquez: "Who Owns My Life?"

"Appeal Court Upholds Exemption from Doctor-Assisted Suicide Ban," *The Canadian Press,* 10 August 2012.
http://www2.macleans.ca/2012/08/10/appeal-court-upholds-exemption-from-doctor-assisted-suicide-ban/

"Assisted Suicide: Canada Revisits An Old Debate," *Associated Press,* Vancouver, 4 December 2011.
http://www.foxnews.com/world/2011/12/04/canada-revisits-old-debate-on-assisted-suicide/

Gyapong, Deborah. "Federal Government Appeals B.C. Decision Striking Down Euthanasia Laws," *Canadian Catholic News,* 14 July 2012. http://www.catholicregister.org/news/canada/item/14880-federal-government-appeals-bc-decision-striking-down-euthanasia-law

Lang, Georgialee. "Euthanasia: A Form of Medical Treatment or Compassionate Murder?" 16 June 2012. http://o.canada.com/2012/06/16/euthanasia-a-form-of-medical-treatment-or-compassionate-murder/

Rodriguez, Sue. "If I cannot give consent to my own death, whose body is this? Who owns my life?" *CBC News: Videotape Presented to Canadian Parliament,* 1992. http://www.cbc.ca/news/canada/the-fight-for-the-right-to-die-1.1130837

Somerville, Margaret. "When is Euthanasia Justified?" *Globe and Mail,* 12 March 2010. http://www.theglobeandmail.com/life/health-and-fitness/when-is-euthanasia-justified/article4392696/

CHAPTER NINE

Dr. Jack Kevorkian: Hero Or Criminal

Chua-Eoan, Howard. "The Life and Deaths of Jack Kevorkian (1928–2011)," *Time,* 3 June 2011.

http://content.time.com/time/nation/article/0,8599,2075644,00.html

Hull, Jon; Kevorkian, Jack. "Kevorkian Speaks His Mind," *Time,* 31 May 1993. http://content.time.com/time/magazine/article/0,9171,978605,00.html

Kevorkian, Jack. *Prescription Medicine: The Goodness of Planned Death.* Prometheus Books, 1991.
http://books.google.com/books/about/Prescription_medicide.html?id=UpHhAAAAMAAJ

Patients' Rights Council: http://www.patientsrightscouncil.org/site/the-real-jack-kevorkian/

"Profile: 'Dr. Death'," *The BBC* (British Broadcasting Corporation), 26 November 1998. http://news.bbc.co.uk/2/hi/americas/222218.stm

CHAPTER TEN

Stairway To Heaven: How To Die In Oregon

Lowe, Justin. "How To Die In Oregon," *Hollywood Reporter,* 28 January 2011. http://www.hollywoodreporter.com/review/sundance-review-hbos-doc-die-89524

Mesh, Aaron. "An Interview with Director Peter Richardson," *Willametter Week,* 17 February 2011.

Richardson, Peter D. (Director, Editor); Snider, Greg, (Co-Editor,) *How To Die In Oregon,* HBO Documentary, 2011. http://www.howtodieinoregon.com

CHAPTER ELEVEN

Oregon, Washington, Montana: Death With Dignity Laws

Death With Dignity National Center: http://www.deathwithdignity.org/

"End-of-Life Practices in the Netherlands under the Euthanasia Act," *New England Journal of Medicine,* May 2007. http://www.nejm.org/doi/full/10.1056/NEJMsa071143

ProCon.org: http://www.euthanasia.procon.org

"Safeguards for 'Death With Dignity' Laws to Ensure that Patients Cannot be Forced, Intimidated, or Coerced into having Doctor-Assisted Death," *Death With Dignity National Center*, Posted by Melissa Barber, 5 April 2011. http://www.deathwithdignity.org/author/melissa-barber

"Twelve Years of Research Data Re: Death With Dignity Legislation." Oregon Department of Human Services, Death With Dignity Statistics - 12 Years. *The Oregon Department of Human Services*, Posted by George Eighmey, 19 January 2011. http://www.deathwithdignity.org/2011/01/19/oregons-law-withstands-test-time

CHAPTER TWELVE

Netherlands, Belgium, Luxembourg: Voluntary Euthanasia Laws

"Assisted suicide rate continues to climb in region of Belgium," *Associated Press,* 9 September 2012.
http://www.oregonlive.com/health/index.ssf/2009/09/assisted_suicide_rate_continue.html

Baklinski, Thaddeus. "Luxembourg Legalizes Euthanasia," 18 March 2009. *http://www.lifesitenews.com/news/archive//ldn/2009/mar/09031803*

"Belgium Euthanasia Cases Jump After New Law: 2002 Ruling Gave Terminally Ill Patients More Options," *Associated Press,* 9 September 2009. *http://www.nbcnews.com/id/32759186/ns/health-health_care/t/belgium-euthanasia-cases-jump-after-new-law/*

Berghmans, Ron L.P.; Widdershoven, Guy A.M. "Euthanasia in the Netherlands: Consultation and Review," *Kings Law Journal,* Volume 23, Number 2, Hart Publishing, August 2012.
http://www.ingentaconnect.com/content/hart/klj/2012/00000023/00000002/art00002

Death With Dignity National Center: *http://www.deathwithdignity.org*

Infoplease: *http://www.infoplease.com/search?q=euthanasia&search=search&fr=iptn*

Kessler, Glenn. "Euthanasia in the Netherlands: Rick Santorum's Bogus Statistics," *Washington Post,* 22 February 2012.
http://www.washingtonpost.com/blogs/fact-checker/post/euthanasia-in-the-netherlands-rick-santorums-bogus-statistics/2012/02/21/gIQAJaRbSR_blog.html

ProCon.org: *http://www.euthanasia.procon.org*

Schadenberg, Alex. "Euthanasia Prevention Coalition," 2009. *LifeSiteNews:* *http://www.lifesitenews.com*

The International Humanist and Ethical Union: Belgium's Legalization of Euthanasia, "Palliative Care/Euthanasia Bill," *Belgium News Bioethics,* 1 February 2003.

CHAPTER THIRTEEN

Switzerland: Tourism Aid In Dying

Button, James. "My name is Dr. John Elliott and I'm about to Die, with my Head Held High," *Sidney Morning Herald,* 26 January 2007. http://www.smh.com.au/articles/2007/01/26/1169788692086.html

Carter v Canada FACTS (Court Document), 2012. "Current Law Regarding Assisted Suicide," *Patients' Rights Council,* Switzerland, 2013. http://www.patientsrightscouncil.org/site/switzerland/

Malarek, Victor. "Seeking an End to Life and Challenging the Law," *CTV News,* 15 October 2011. http://www.ctvnews.ca/w5-seeking-an-end-to-life-and-challenging-the-law-1.711234

The Swiss Model: http://www.exitinternational.net/page/Switzerland

CHAPTER FOURTEEN

Gloria Taylor: "Personal Exemption" For Physician - Assisted Death

"A B.C. Supreme Court Judge has Struck Down Canada's Ban on Doctor-Assisted Suicide as Unconstitutional," *The Province,* 1 December 2011. http://www.chat-avenue.com/forums/showthread.php?201355-BC-judge-rules-law-banning-doctor-assisted-suicide-uncons

"Appeals Court Upholds Exemption from Doctor-Assisted Suicide Ban," *Canadian Press,* 10 August 2012. http://www2.macleans.ca/2012/08/10/appeal-court-upholds-exemption-from-doctor-assisted-suicide-ban/

"Assisted Suicide: Canada Revisits An Old Debate," *Associated Press,* Vancouver, 4 December 2011. http://www.foxnews.com/world/2011/12/04/canada-revisits-old-debate-on-assisted-suicide/

Carter v Canada (Attorney General) (2012): BC Court Rules that Ban on Assisted Suicide is Unconstitutional: Author: Leah McDaniel. 7 August 2012.

"Court Upholds B.C. Woman's Exemption from Doctor-Assisted Suicide Ban," *Canadian Press* - Vancouver, 10 August 2012.
http://www.theglobeandmail.com/news/british-columbia/court-upholds-bc-womans-exemption-from-doctor-assisted-suicide-ban/article4474112/

Doctor-Assisted Suicide Ban," *Canadian Press* - Vancouver, 10 August 2012.

Dhillon, Sunny. "B.C. Civil Liberties Group Sues to Legalize Euthanasia in Canada," *Globe and Mail*, 14 November 2011.
http://www.theglobeandmail.com/life/health-and-fitness/bc-civil-liberties-group-sues-to-legalize-euthanasia-in-canada/article4200469/

"Gloria Taylor Dead: Euthanasia Crusader Dies Of Infection," *Huffington Post*, B.C., 5 October 2012.
http://www.huffingtonpost.ca/2012/10/05/gloria-taylor-dead-euthanasia-right-to-die-assisted-suicide_n_1944219.html

Gyapong, Deborah. "Federal Government Appeals B.C. Decision Striking Down Euthanasia Laws," *Canadian Catholic News*, 14 July 2012. http://www.catholicregister.org/news/canada/item/14880-federal-government-appeals-bc-decision-striking-down-euthanasia-laws

Hume, Mark. "Government Lawyer Draws Line Between Euthanasia and War," *Globe and Mail*, 8 December 2011.
http://www.theglobeandmail.com/life/health-and-fitness/government-lawyer-draws-line-between-euthanasia-and-war/article4247245/

Keller, James. "Judge Upholds Gloria Taylor's Right to Die," *Canadian Press*, 11 August 2012.
http://www.canada.com/vancouversun/news/westcoastnews/story.html?id=c0d774c7-ef65-470a-b29c-3bcd5ce1b64a

Lang, Georgialee. "Euthanasia: A Form of Medical Treatment or Compassionate Murder?" 16 June 2012.
http://o.canada.com/2012/06/16/euthanasia-a-form-of-medical-treatment-or-compassionate-murder/

Malarek, Victor. "Seeking an End to Life and Challenging the Law," *CTV News*, 15 October 2011. http://www.ctvnews.ca/w5-seeking-an-end-to-life-and-challenging-the-law-1.711234

Rodriguez, Sue. "If I cannot give consent to my own death, whose body is this? Who owns my life?" *CBC News: Videotape Presented to Canadian Parliament,* 1992. http://www.cbc.ca/news/canada/the-fight-for-the-right-to-die-1.1130837

Somerville, Margaret. "When Is Euthanasia Justified?" *Globe and Mail,* 12 March 2010. http://www.theglobeandmail.com/life/health-and-fitness/when-is-euthanasia-justified/article4392696/

Verma, Sonia. "Mercy-killing Debate is Back with a Vengeance," *Globe and Mail,* 14 November 2011.
http://www.theglobeandmail.com/life/health-and-fitness/mercy-killing-debate-is-back-with-a-vengeance/article4200472/

Worthington, Peter. "Dying with Dignity: Trust Our Doctors," *QMI Agency,* 29 January 2012. http://www.torontosun.com/2012/01/27/dying-with-dignity-trust-our-doctors

CHAPTER FIFTEEN

Tony Nicklinson: The Trapped Man

"Anna Soubry, Britain's Newly-Appointed Health Minister, Declared that Britain's Laws on Assisted-Death Needed to Change," *Huffington Press Association,* 9 August 2012.
http://www.huffingtonpost.co.uk/2012/09/08/health-minister-anna-soubry-suicide-laws_n_1866749.html

"Assisted Dying Debate: Tony Nicklinson in his Own Words," *BBC News,* 19 June 2012. http://www.bbc.com/news/uk-england-wiltshire-18398797#http://www.bbc.co.uk/news/uk-england-wiltshire-18398797%20

Gregory, Andrew. "Locked-in Syndrome Sufferer Tony Nicklinson Breaks Down as High Court Rejects Right-to-Die Bid," *The Times Co. UK,* 17 August 2012. http://www.dailyrecord.co.uk/news/uk-world-news/tony-nicklinson-loses-court-bid-1265288

"'Let my husband die': Locked-in syndrome sufferer wins High Court hearing for his right-to-die after wife's legal bid: Businessman Tony Nicklinson wants Judge to end his 'Indignity' following Stroke in 2005," *Mirror News,* 3 March 2012.
http://www.mirror.co.uk/news/uk-news/let-my-husband-die-locked-in-syndrome-759160

"Right-to-Die Man Tony Nicklinson Dead after Refusing Food," *BBC News*, 22 August 2012. *http://www.bbc.co.uk/news/uk-england-19341722*

Stone, Lee. "Tony Nicklinson: The Trapped Man," *BBC Wiltshire*, 22 August 2012. *http://www.bbc.co.uk/news/uk-england-wiltshire-19348267*

"Tony Nicklinson: Funeral of 'Right-to-Die' Campaigner Held," *BBC News,* 31 August 2012. *http://www.bbc.co.uk/news/uk-england-wiltshire-19442966*

CHAPTER SIXTEEN

Massachusetts 2012: Physician Aid In Dying Ballot Fails

Saunders, Dr. Peter. "Defeat for Pro-Euthanasia Lobby as Massachusetts Rejects Assisted Suicide on Ballot," *National Right-to-Life News,* 8 November 2012.
http://www.nationalrighttolifenews.org/news/2012/11/defeat-for-pro-euthanasia-lobby-as-massachusetts-rejects-assisted-suicide-on-ballot/#.UjfdYhY-ZGE

Schadenberg, Alex. "Do Americans Want to Legalize Assisted Suicide?" *National Right-to-Life News,* 3 January 2013.
http://www.nationalrighttolifenews.org/news/2013/01/do-americans-want-to-legalize-assisted-suicide/#more-20812

CHAPTER SEVENTEEN

To Gently Leave This Life

"Belgium Euthanasia Cases Jump After New Law: 2002 Ruling Gave Terminally Ill Patients More Options," *Associated Press,* 9 September 2009. *http://www.nbcnews.com/id/32759186/ns/health-health_care/t/belgium-euthanasia-cases-jump-after-new-law/#.UjfeBhY-ZGE*

Brasil, Luiz. "Bill 52 Could Make Quebec the First Province to Legalize Euthanasia," *The Brock Press*, 4 March 2014. *http://www.brockpress.com/2014/03/bill-52-could-make-quebec-the-first-province-to-legalize-euthanasia/*

Eckholm, Erik."Aid in Dying Movement Takes Hold in Some States," *New York Times*, 7 February 2014.
http://www.nytimes.com/2014/02/08/us/easing-terminal-patients-path-to-death-legally.html

PHOTOGRAPHS

Kaplan, Larry. Photo Enhancements: *To Gently Leave This Life*, September 2013.

10676731R00069

Made in the USA
San Bernardino, CA
23 April 2014